Handbook of Primate Husbandry and Welfare

Handbook of Primate Husbandry and Welfare

Sarah Wolfensohn

BSc, MA, VetMB, Cert LAS, CBiol, FIBiol, Dip ECLAM, MRCVS
Head of Department, Veterinary Services, University of Oxford

and

Paul Honess

BSc, PhD
Research Primatologist
Veterinary Services, University of Oxford

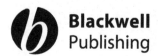

Blackwell Publishing

Editorial Offices:
Blackwell Publishing Ltd, 9600 Garsington Road, Oxford OX4 2DQ, UK
  Tel: +44 (0)1865 776868
Blackwell Publishing Professional, 2121 State Avenue, Ames, Iowa 50014-8300, USA
  Tel: +1 515 292 0140
Blackwell Publishing Asia Pty Ltd, 550 Swanston Street, Carlton, Victoria 3053, Australia
  Tel: +61 (0)3 8359 1011

First published 2005 by Blackwell Publishing Ltd

Library of Congress Cataloging-in-Publication Data
Wolfensohn, Sarah.
  Handbook of primate husbandry and welfare/Sarah Wolfensohn and
  Paul Honess. — 1st ed.
     p.   cm.
  Includes bibliographical references and index.
  ISBN 1–4051–1158–5 (pbk. : alk. paper)
  1. Primates as laboratory animals.   2. Captive wild animals.   3. Animal welfare.
  I. Honess, Paul.   II. Title.

  SF407.P7W66 2005
  636.98—dc22

                                                                    2004010531
  ISBN 1–4051–1158–5

A catalogue record for this title is available from the British Library

Set in 10/12.5 Times
by Integra Software Services Pvt. Ltd, Pondicherry, India

The publisher's policy is to use permanent paper from mills that operate a sustainable
forestry policy, and which has been manufactured from pulp processed using acid-free
and elementary chlorine-free practices. Furthermore, the publisher ensures that the text
paper and cover board used have met acceptable environmental accreditation standards.

For further information on Blackwell Publishing, visit our website:
www.blackwellpublishing.com

Contents

Preface

All animals should receive good husbandry and welfare but, because of their close phylogenetic relationship to man, primates are often given special status. Primates are intelligent and responsive, and working with them can be extremely rewarding. The authors do not believe that primates have specific rights; but that we, as their keepers, have a duty to ensure that their lives are as comfortable as possible and that the five freedoms are adhered to. That is:

- freedom from thirst, hunger or malnutrition
- freedom from discomfort
- freedom from pain, injury and disease
- freedom to express normal behaviour
- freedom from fear and distress.

These five freedoms are taken from the UK Farm Animal Welfare Council recommendations, yet they are even more applicable to a creature that has greater capacity for psychological suffering by isolation, boredom and restriction of movement than a farm animal, and so should be even more rigorously applied to primates.

If the use of primates in research facilities, zoos, or private collections is to be supported there is an ethical obligation to house and maintain them in the best conditions that can be provided, so as 'best practice' evolves it is necessary to continually question if the facilities and their operation and management can be improved. While a good deal is known about the needs of primates in captivity, there are a number of aspects where more scientifically validated information would be welcome to supplement the experience on which the present recommendations are largely based.

The purpose of this book is to encourage discussion and active review of the husbandry of captive primates and to assist with the management of changes to benefit their welfare. The authors' experience covers both wild and captive primates and currently they both work with primates kept for laboratory use. Although this is reflected in many of the examples given to illustrate the points made, the principles of improving primate welfare can be applied to all captive primates whether in zoos, laboratories or private collections. Whatever the purpose for keeping a primate it will need to be housed and cared for, diseases will need to be prevented and health and safety issues of those caring for it will need to be addressed. Some of the discussion is deliberately contentious; there are not platitudes to keep the majority content, but it seeks to sow the seeds of discontent in some current methodologies in order to stimulate progression toward a better future for these species whose lives enrich ours – either by contributing to progress in the fight against disease, allowing us the opportunity to observe and learn from their behaviour, or by providing us with more diverse fauna.

Acknowledgements

We are indebted to our colleagues at Oxford University Veterinary Services for their support and encouragement throughout the writing of this book, particularly Paul Finnemore. We are also grateful to the management at Harlan UK who have provided financial support for our research work and to their staff for assistance, particularly Tony Brown. Graham Tobin provided a significant contribution to Chapter 4 and Phyllis Lee gave valuable guidance on Chapter 8.

Cover photo by Paul Honess. Additional photos have been supplied by Harlan UK, Oxford University Biomedical Services Department, Simon Bearder, Centre for Macaques and BFC Farm, Israel for which we are grateful.

This book is dedicated to Gringo whose gentle nature encouraged us to develop better methods of husbandry, from which his offspring will benefit.

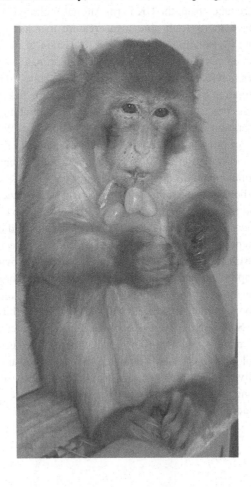

Chapter 1
Primates: Their characteristics and relationship with man

WHAT IS A PRIMATE?

Primates are one of 18 orders within the Class Mammalia (mammals). Primates are an arboreal adapted group found in a wide range of arboreal and some non-arboreal habitats across the tropical areas of the world and extending into some subtropical and temperate areas (see Figure 1.1). When the modern distribution of humans is taken into account it is clear that primates, as a group, have colonised almost all terrestrial habitats on Earth, including extreme deserts and polar regions. There are over 200 species of primate divided into two sub-orders; the Haplorhini (the haplorhines: tarsiers, monkeys, apes and humans) and the Strepsirhini (the strepsirhines: bushbabies, lorises and lemurs). They range in body size from approximately 35 g (mouse lemur) to over 170 kg (adult male gorilla).

A simplified illustration of the classification of living primates can be seen in Figure 1.2 (see Groves, 2001 for a detailed treatment of primate taxonomy). This is the order to which man and his very closest relatives belong. This relationship has profound implications for the other members of this group, both in terms of our study of our relatives as a way to understand more about ourselves, and the limits that are placed on that study by ethical judgements on the nature and extent of those studies.

Of great importance when considering these matters is to have a clear perspective of not only the characteristics that we share with our non-human primate (hereafter referred to simply as primate) relatives but also those features that make us different from them.

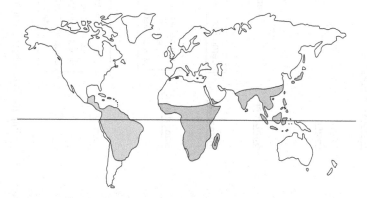

Figure 1.1   A map showing the distribution of wild primates.

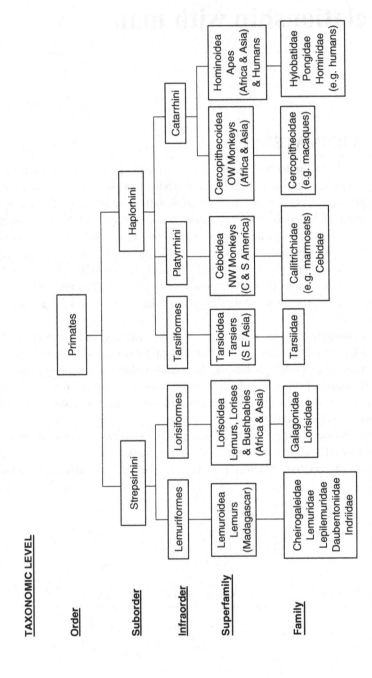

Figure 1.2   A simplified classification of living primates.

PRIMATE CHARACTERISTICS

Primates are unusual among mammal groups as there is no all-inclusive definition that defines them as an order (Martin 1990). Instead a number of general trends can be identified among the members of this group, although exceptions exist in many instances. Some authors have summarised what it is to be a primate:

It has, in fact, been a common theme throughout the literature on primate evolution that primates lack any clear-cut diagnostic features of the kind found in other placental mammals.

Martin (1990)

If there is an essence of being a primate it is the progressive evolution of intelligence as a way of life.

Jolly (1985)

Primates have an evolutionary origin over 70 million years ago and although living representatives of this group can be found in tropical and subtropical arboreal habitats in Africa, Asia and Central and South America, fossil forms had a much more extensive distribution which included North America and Europe (Martin 1990; Fleagle 1999).

Of perhaps greatest importance are the large brains that primates have relative to their body weight. These large brains, while placing a significant energetic burden on the animal, allow expansion in areas of integration, perception and manipulation as well as enabling complex social behaviour and specifically the management of social relationships (for an overview of primate sociality, social and breeding systems see Chapters 7 and 8). Primate infants have a long period of dependence on their mother during which they learn vital elements of what is and isn't appropriate to eat as well as issues of social etiquette. Primates have a late first age of reproduction and produce small litter sizes (typically one) and at extended inter-litter intervals to allow primate parents to make the required investment in their offsprings' slow development.

As a group primates are well-adapted to a climbing, leaping, arboreal life; they are hind-limb dominated giving them a posterior centre of gravity. Although there are a few exceptions, primates typically have five digits on grasping hands and feet, with opposable thumbs and big toes. Some species have secondarily evolved claws although most have nails and all primates have at least one nail, on the big toe. These nails support gripping fleshy pads containing pressure-sensitive Meissner's corpuscles that contribute to the fine sense of touch that primates have. Also, primates can be seen to have a rather generalised dentition that does not show the type of specialisation for food handling and processing seen among other groups of mammals with specialised diets (e.g. specialist herbivores and insectivores). This reflects a generalised diet in primates.

Despite their good sense of touch, high dexterity and a keen sense of smell, retained from the ancestral mammal, primates, sensory emphasis is visual. Their forward-facing eyes and highly developed visual centres in the brain are associated with the three dimensional, stereoscopic, colour vision that primates have.

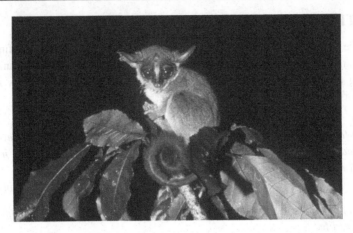

Figure 1.3 The rondo dwarf galago (*Galagoides rondoensis*): a typical strepsirhine and among the smallest living primates, at around 50 g.

The strepsirhines

The strepsirhines, restricted to Africa, Madagascar and tropical Asia, represent those living primates that most closely resemble the first primates that appear in the fossil record about 55 million years ago (Figure 1.3). They are predominantly, with the exception of some of the lemur species, nocturnal with a suite of anatomical and behavioural characteristics best suited to their nocturnal lifestyle. Their sensory emphasis follows this pattern and includes large light-gathering eyes with a reflective tapetum behind the retina and poor or non-existent colour vision. They have large, often independently moveable ears, a well-developed sense of smell and chemoreception via a moist, naked nasal rhinarium and vomeronasal organ. The canines and incisors in the lower jaw are formed into a 'toothcomb'. Despite having some of the smallest brains for their body size among the primates, many species of strepsirhines, whilst being solitary foragers, nevertheless live socially complex lives, managing social relationships with those with whom they have overlapping ranges and with whom they may share sleeping sites. Much communication takes place at a spatial or temporal distance via the media of vocal and olfactory communication.

The haplorhines

The haplorhines are found across the tropics, with the exception of the strepsirhine stronghold of Madagascar. They are, with the exception of the tarsiers (*Tarsius* spp.) and owl monkeys (*Aotus* spp.), diurnal and characterised by their refined visual sense, particularly their colour vision, and their complex social organisation (Figure 1.4). Substantial differences exist between the major groups within the haplorhines: the tarsiers (South-east Asia), New World monkeys (Central and South America), Old World monkeys (Africa and Asia), apes (Africa and South-east Asia) and humans (worldwide). Hence generalised characteristics are seen in brain expansion compared with strepsirhines, post-orbital bony

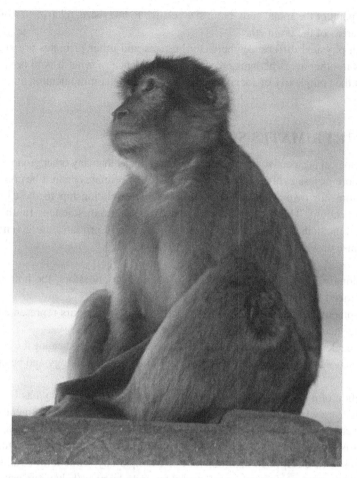

Figure 1.4   The Barbary macaque (*Macaca sylvanus*) native to the cedar forests of Morocco and Algeria. An introduced population in Gibraltar represents Europe's only primate species.

closure, nails rather than claws (except tarsiers and the small New World callitrichid primates) as well as the presence of sexual cycles and specialised placental structure.

Human–primate differences

Human beings (*Homo sapiens*), however, are very different from other primates in a range of ways and this is covered by many authors of texts on human/primate evolution (e.g. Martin 1990; Tattersall 1998; Fleagle 1999). Many of the skeletal differences derive from changes due to the development of a novel primate locomotory style: bipedalism. Major differences can be seen between humans and other primates in the structure of the foot, the knee and the hip as well as the shape of the spine and the position of the skull on the spine. These reflect engineering solutions that both allow bipedalism and make it an efficient mode of locomotion. The skull houses many of the most important differences between humans and other primates including: jaw shape, degree of prognathism, cranial shape, exit point of the spinal cord, brain size relative to body size, relative size of different functional areas of the brain etc.

Although physical differences between humans and other primates are substantial, differences in other areas perhaps provide more evidence of what it is to be human, for example in the complexity of social behaviour, cognition, communication and the use of technology.

WHY ARE PRIMATES SPECIAL?

From a zoological perspective primates are no more special than any other group of animals, being no more or less evolved. However, the status of primates cannot be considered in isolation from our own when our close phylogenetic relationship to these animals is taken into account. Therefore when viewed from a human sciences (anthropology, psychology, medicine etc.) or anthropocentric perspective primates are given a special status because of what we can learn from them by studying:

- evolutionary history, including what our own direct ancestors, the hominids, may have looked and behaved like – how we got where we are;
- developmental aspects of structures, processes and behaviours represented in other primate species;
- adaptive relevance of structures, processes and behaviours; understanding the evolutionary and functional significance of aspects of our anatomy, physiology and behaviour.

Exploration of a number of these areas in primates, when homology has been conclusively demonstrated, can contribute to the investigation and possible treatment of disease and dysfunction in humans. This raises the issue of the study of primates as a model for humans. It is clear that the validity of the primate model has more serious implications for some research disciplines than others. For example any reduction in validity of the study of wild or captive chimpanzees as a model for proto-humans (behaviour, psychology or ecology) would be likely to have less serious implications than if the macaque model currently in use in neuroscience, toxicology and immunology studies were invalid. The choice of a species as the nearest best model may still not mean it is a *good enough* model of humans. Some of the history and ethical debate surrounding this contentious issue will be discussed later in this chapter.

The basis for special consideration for primates, in terms of regulatory oversight of studies involving primates, stems not just from emotive aspects of our ability to empathise best with our closest relatives and to anthropomorphise about them, their treatment and their plight, but also from objective consideration of their ability to feel pain and to suffer. The large brain for their size that primates have, their sophisticated cognitive abilities and their high reliance on sociality and complex social systems lead us to believe that their perception of pain as well as cognitive and social deprivation may not be so different from our own. Over the last 20–30 years there has been a gradual shifting of the goal-posts on views on what separates us from our primate relatives. From tool-use and manufacture (Goodall 1964) through to the use of symbolism in communication (Savage-Rumbaugh 1992), more extensive and long-term studies of primates continue to erode these barriers to humanness. Despite a genetic distance of less than 2% between humans and chimpanzees there remain substantial differences between humans and apes even to the casual observer. Dogs, for example share about 75% of their genetic material with humans yet have few apparent similarities.

Human rights for apes?

With the reduction of the conceptual gap between humans and particularly the members of the great apes, it is inevitable that many will begin to call for an extension of all or some human rights to these species. Your view on this matter may well be influenced by whether you believe that the reduction of differences between humans and the great apes results in us moving closer to them, or them being elevated closer to us.

There are moves among some to classify humans and certain of the great apes, particularly the chimpanzee, together, including suggestions of extending the genus *Homo* to include these species. This however is problematic as not only would it defy the stark morphological differences between humans and the other apes, but it would also create a problem in deciding which species to exclude. For example, while including the other great apes, would there be basis for excluding gorillas (*Gorilla gorilla*)? They may not be as cognitively sophisticated as chimpanzees (*Pan troglodytes*), bonobos (*P. paniscus*) or, of course, humans, but these ape species have a much greater degree of similarity in their morphology, behaviour and ecology with each other than any of them have with humans.

The implication of recent calls for the extension of human rights to apes would be far-reaching, not only for long-established beliefs about mankind's place in the natural world, but also for treatment of his primate relatives including the continued maintenance of these species in any form of captivity as research subjects, zoo exhibits or as pets. If the apes were given this special consideration it would become increasingly difficult to justify any such treatment of *any* species of primate. A possible alternative, that addresses a number of concerns, is to recognise the biological similarity and shared evolutionary history of humans and our closest relatives and redouble efforts to treat them more as collaborators, rather than animate pieces of laboratory equipment, in our efforts to resolve many of the most important health challenges we face. Optimised welfare is an essential element of this; increasing public pressure and empirical evidence make a strong moral and scientific case for striving beyond the simple physiological maintenance of these 'animate pieces of laboratory equipment' towards a welfare intensive collaboration. Carried out correctly this will produce more psychologically and physiologically natural and accurate models and, thereby, better science. A strong emphasis through regulation and grant funding on the 3Rs (Reduction, Refinement and Replacement; Russell & Birch 1959) may enable researchers to work towards the eventual redundancy of primate individuals in research programmes with the development of alternatives (e.g. *in vitro* and computer-based models) that more accurately predict human biology.

World Heritage status

While animal rights sentiment may be the prime motivating force for the campaign for the extension of human rights to the apes, other moves are under way, which have their origin among conservationists, that would have a considerable impact on the status of the apes and, perhaps in the future, other primate or indeed other animal species. This is the move to have members of the great apes declared World Heritage Species. It is, rightly, believed that this would add significantly to the profile of these species and their conservation plight in the wild. Moves calling for this special status for these species are currently beset by the political issue of large numbers of apes, primarily chimpanzees, continuing to be maintained in the USA for research projects. Compromise moves for this status to be granted only to those individuals of these species in the wild may well be viewed as nonsensical by the public and hence any impact of awarding this status may be lost.

ETHICAL CONSIDERATIONS OF ANIMALS IN CAPTIVITY

Mankind has a long history of association with animals from commensal to the earliest domestication, whether this be for utility, food or companionship/curiosity (Clutton-Brock 1999). The last 200 years has seen a significant increase in the numbers of animals maintained in captivity in all these categories, but it is only relatively recently that ethical considerations relating to the treatment of animals have been enshrined in law.

However, it has been advances in medical science and product testing (including pharmaceutical products) that have resulted in the substantial numbers of primates maintained in captivity. Simultaneously there are increasing concerns in society about how animals are maintained in captivity and to what use they are put. While there is still room for considerable improvement in many cases, there have been revolutions since the 1970s in the standards of animal care in the best zoos and research establishments. However it is now well established that, where there is a justification to keep animals in captivity, it is a duty of those that keep them to ensure that they are kept in conditions that address their health and welfare requirements. With animals such as primates this can involve considerable cost; both in terms of veterinary attention, environmental conditions and suitable and specific social and environmental enrichment (see Chapter 6). For these reasons primates do not make suitable pets and professional societies of primatologists do not recommend them as such.

Primates, particularly chimpanzees and orang-utans have historically been used in television advertising and as exhibits in circuses. Both of these uses, which frequently involve dressing the animals in clothes and making them behave like humans, are becoming rarer. While some may feel that such use of these animals helps elevate their profile in the public consciousness and in some instances may be educational, others feel strongly that such use demeans these creatures and fosters inappropriate attitudes towards them, such as excessive anthropomorphism. It is true that things can be learnt from the training of these primates to perform which may be transferable, for example training primates to cooperate with husbandry and other procedures in different contexts where primates are kept in captivity. However caution must be exercised as not all training techniques are acceptable as evidenced when circus trainer Mary Chipperfield was found guilty in the UK in 1999 of animal cruelty under the Protection of Animals Act (1911) after being secretly filmed repeatedly beating a number of animals including a young chimpanzee (http:/ /news.bbc.co.uk/1/hi/uk/263864.stm).

The justification for keeping primates, as many other species, in zoos has shifted away from curiosity and entertainment to recognising their value in conservation education and also as suitable flagship species in captive breeding programmes. Arguments continue about the relative merits of *in situ* (in habitat and range countries) and *ex situ* (non-habitat or non-range countries) breeding programmes. Where the target species is in less imminent risk of extinction *in situ* programmes may be preferable, whereas with highest risk species that may require specialist action (including assisted reproduction) or in instances where no natural habitat remains, *ex situ* programmes may be necessary.

A number of factors relating to their slow reproductive turnover, their sensitivity to disturbance, in many cases their degree of ecological specialisation and, not least, their visibility and audibility, make primates excellent candidates as indicator species for ecological surveys aiming to examine the conservation status and health of an ecosystem. The same reasons, coupled with their high reliance on social stimulus from conspecifics, high level of curiosity and low boredom threshold also make primates difficult to maintain *optimally* in captivity. Meeting all their social, behavioural, ecological and environmental needs presents significant challenges to carers of primates, if animals are to be maintained in a physically and psychologically healthy condition.

Of increasing importance is the role of sanctuaries. Many in the developed world focus on the rescue of primates that have been confiscated as pets owing to poor welfare standards, or as victims of the illegal trafficking for the pet or zoo trade. Sanctuaries established in habitat countries care for those orphaned or injured as a result of environmental disasters, as in the case of orang-utans with the continued deforestation and the catastrophic forest fires in Indonesia in the late 1990s, or as casualties of the continuing bushmeat trade which threatens many populations of primates in West and Central Africa (Cowlishaw & Dunbar 2000; Fa *et al.* 2002). In instances where it is not possible or desirable to reintroduce these animals to the wild, sanctuaries perform a vital role in providing a safe alternative. A few sanctuaries will also re-house zoo exhibits that are old, injured or experience behavioural problems and only a very few will take into retirement primates from experimental institutions, including those that have been the subject of neuroscience research. Many increasingly believe that more effort should be made to retire ex-experimental primates, including a large number of ex-HIV-study apes in the USA (Strier 2000), into sanctuaries with the highest welfare standards and under strict conditions of confidentiality. It should, of course, be pointed out that wild primate populations are not always accorded such protection. As human populations expand and make greater demands on natural resources they are pushed into competitive interactions with many species of wildlife, whose natural habitat may be being eroded by agricultural and other developmental activity. In these instances wildlife can come to be regarded as pests; the classic example is that of crop-raiding, which in many tropical areas can involve primates. In Africa common problem species include baboons (*Papio* spp.) and vervet monkeys (*Cercopithecus aethiops*), which are widespread and generally not under conservation threat and in some instances culling programmes may be seen as a control option. In parts of South-east Asia some relatively common species like the long-tailed macaque, *Macaca fascicularis* (also known as the cynomolgus or crab-eating macaque, but referred to throughout this book as the long-tailed macaque) are also considered pests. A unique challenge is presented in some parts of the world, for example in Sulawesi, where macaque species that are locally abundant and considered agricultural pests, have very limited distribution and are therefore considered to have high conservation threat status.

Cultural considerations

Naturally there are cross-cultural differences in the way that societies view their relationship with other animals, including primates. An example of this can be found in the consumption and trading of primates for food, both in areas of West and Central Africa (the 'bushmeat trade') and in parts of South-east Asia and the Far East. In that context it is perhaps unrealistic to expect the treatment of primates in these regions to be the same as in those areas where ethical values are derived from a Judeo-Christian tradition of stewardship of animals. It, at least in part, explains different levels of regulation and enforcement of regulation seen in different countries. This has implications particularly for the examination of housing and welfare conditions in primate breeding centres in these regions that may be used as sources of primates for scientific use. However, commercial pressures are valuable in encouraging reform in conditions which may not be achieved through ethical arguments. Overseas breeding of primates is examined at greater length in Chapter 9. Differences also exist between developed Western nations in the exercise of ethical oversight of the use of animals in science. In some instances this is left to the discretion of individual establishments, within general guidelines (e.g. USA), in others there are more rigorous structures such as those found in the UK. In the UK, the combination of the local Ethical Review Process, Home Office licensing, the Animal Procedures Committee and possibly the strictest animal protection legislation in the world (The Animal (Scientific Procedures) Act (1986)), provides arguably the toughest central oversight and accountability in the world. With this degree of oversight and accountability, it is inevitable that such measures will be viewed as overly bureaucratic and restrictive by many researchers. Potentially this may have the effect of forcing some researchers to move their research programmes to other countries where there are fewer restrictions on the type of research they wish to conduct. This remains unavoidable in the context of public, and thereby political opinion, being intolerant of what it may regard as overly invasive or ethically questionable research.

Even among professional primatologists some broad cultural differences can be seen in the underlying approach to the study of primate behaviour, particularly social behaviour. This can be most clearly seen between Japanese and Western primatologists. Western primatologists focus on the study of populations frequently to elucidate species-typical patterns of behaviour, whereas there has been a history among Japanese primatologists of studying primate social behaviour in the context of the interaction of interindividual relationships and personalities in determining the character and nature of social behaviour within a social unit (Asquith 1986). The Japanese approach has often been viewed by Western researchers as overly anthropomorphic and lacking the objectivity that is so highly valued in Western scientific tradition.

LEGAL CONSIDERATIONS

United States of America

The main federal legislation in the USA that governs the use of animals in science is the Animal Welfare Act (1966), its amendments and associated legislation. Inspection of facilities to ensure compliance with the legislation is carried out by US Department of Agriculture rather than the National Institutes of Health (NIH) through whom much of the funding for animal, particularly primate-using, research is sourced. Additional state legislation governing the use and welfare of animals exists that requires specific, local compliance. Guidelines for institutions and individuals conducting primate-based research are laid out in the *Guide for the Care and Use of Laboratory Animals* produced by the National Research Council and published by the National Academy Press (NRC, 1996). This volume includes guidance in several areas:

- the responsibilities and policies of the animal-using institution, laying out the role, composition and the function of the Institutional Animal Care and Use Committee (IACUC) – the Guide also covers the area of protocols for 'animal care and use, occupational health and safety, and personnel qualifications';
- provision of the physical, behavioural and social environment for animals together with husbandry and management guidance and includes *Recommendations* of space provision;
- animal health and veterinary care;
- the design and structure of animal holding and research facilities.

The Guide deals primarily with general issues and principles and despite its widespread use, does not attempt to give details of individual species' requirements and biology, such as may be found in other texts (e.g. Poole 1999).

United Kingdom

The UK is judged to have among the strictest regulations governing the use, care and welfare of animals in science. The cornerstone of the regulations is the Animal (Scientific Procedures) Act (1986). The regulations require all research that involves carrying out procedures for a scientific purpose, which has the potential to cause pain, suffering, distress or lasting harm, on animals (primarily vertebrates) to be conducted only under a project licence granted by the Home Office and by researchers that hold a Home Office personal licence at a site specified on a Certificate of Designation. Detailed, species-specific, *minimum* requirements for housing, health and welfare are laid out in Home Office regulations. These are detailed and placed in a legislative context in Wolfensohn and Lloyd (2003). Compliance with the regulations is overseen by a system of Home Office Inspectors, who advise on the issuing of licences and who also retain the power to suspend licences in the instance of infringement. Special justification is required when applying for a Project Licence for research involving primates and additional justification is necessary for the use of Old World as opposed to New World primates.

European Union

There are moves to harmonise certain areas of animal use governance within the European Union. Regulations governing the use and care of laboratory primates vary considerably across the member states of the European Union and attempts to harmonise policy in this area, as with some other areas of policy in the EU, have proved difficult. Where agreement has been reached it seems that consistency of enforcement still provides a substantial hurdle to true harmonisation across the EU.

Directive 86/609/EEC was adopted by the Council of Europe in 1986; European Convention for the Protection of Vertebrate Animals Used for Experimental and Scientific Purposes (European Treaty Series No. 123 (ETS 123)) aimed to set minimum standards in the housing and care of experimental animals and to improve controls on their use. More recently in 2002 the Scientific Steering Committee of the Health and Consumer Protection Directorate-General produced a report for the European Commission: *The Need for Non-human Primates in Biomedical Research*, which makes recommendations about the maintenance of primates in captivity for research as well as dealing with many of the general issues surrounding the use of primates in research. The report particularly stresses the need to coordinate research across Europe to avoid wasteful duplication of research conducted in different member states.

FURTHER READING

Asquith, P.J. (1986) Anthropomorphism and the Japanese and Western traditions in primatology. In: *Primate Ontogeny Cognition and Social Behaviour.* (eds J.G. Else & P.C. Lee), pp. 61–71. Cambridge University Press, Cambridge.

Blum, D. (1994) *Monkey Wars.* Oxford University Press, Oxford.

Blum, D. (2003) *Love at Goon Park: Harry Harlow and the Science of Affection.* John Wiley, Chichester, UK.

Clutton-Brock, J. (1999) *A Natural History of Domesticated Mammals*, 2nd edn. Cambridge University Press, Cambridge.

Cowlishaw, G. & Dunbar, R.I.M. (2000) *Primate Conservation Biology.* Chicago University Press, Chicago.

European Commission (1986) European Convention for the Protection of Vertebrate Animals Used for Experimental and Scientific Purposes (European Treaty Series No. 123 (ETS 123)). EC, Strasbourg.

Fa, J.E., Peres, C.A. & Meeuwig, J. (2002) Bushmeat exploitation in tropical forests: an intercontinental comparison. *Conservation Biology*, **16** (1), 232–237.

Fleagle, J.G. (1999) *Primate Adaptation and Evolution*, 2nd edn. Academic Press, San Diego, California.

Goodall, J. (1964) Tool-using and aimed throwing in a community of free-living chimpanzees. *Nature*, **201**, 1264–1266.

Groves, C. (2001) *Primate Taxonomy.* Smithsonian Series in Comparative Evolutionary Biology. Smithsonian Institution Press, Washington D.C.

The Home Office. *Animal (Scientific Procedures) Act (1986).* HMSO, London.

Jolly, A. (1985) *The Evolution of Primate Behaviour*, 2nd edn. p. 5. Macmillan, New York.

Martin, R.D. (1990) *Primate Origins and Evolution.* Academic Press, New York.

NRC (1996) *Guide for the Care and Use of Laboratory Animals.* National Research Council. National Academy Press, Washington D.C.

Poole, T.B. (ed.) (1999) *The UFAW Handbook on the Care and Management of Laboratory Animals*, 7th edn. Blackwell Science, Oxford.

Russell, W.M.S. & Birch, R.L. (1959) *The Principles of Humane Experimental Technique: History, Science and Ethics*. Special edition, Universities Federation for Animal Welfare, UK, 1992.

Savage-Rumbaugh, S. (1992) The brain and language: Language training of apes. In: *The Cambridge Encylopaedia of Human Evolution*. (eds S. Jones, R.D. Martin, D. Philbeam), pp. 138–142. Cambridge University Press, Cambridge.

Scientific Steering Committee (Health and Consumer Protection Directorate-General) (2002) *The Need for Non-human Primates in Biomedical Research*. Report for the European Commission, Strasbourg. http://europa.eu.int/comm/food/fs/sc/ssc/out 253_en.pdf

Strier, K.B. (2000) *Primate Behavioural Ecology*. Allyn and Bacon, Boston, Massachusetts.

Tattersall, I. (1998) *Becoming Human: Evolution and Human Uniqueness*. Oxford University Press, Oxford.

Wolfensohn, S.E. & Lloyd, M. (2003) *Handbook of Laboratory Animal Management and Welfare*, 3rd edn. Blackwell Science, Oxford.

Chapter 2
The physical environment

The physical environment in which captive primates are housed is an essential element of the suite of conditions that contribute to the physical and psychological health of the animals.

CONSIDERATIONS IN ACCOMMODATION DESIGN

When designing accommodation in which to keep captive primates, whether for research purposes in zoos or in laboratories or as pets, the starting point is to examine the ecological requirements of the particular species and consider where it lives in the wild and which features of that environment can be reproduced in the captive setting. Not all features of the wild environment are in the animal's welfare interest; for example, food resources may be scarce and competition from conspecifics may be high in the wild, but in the captive setting this is reversed by plentiful provision of food and lower animal stocking densities. However, this may reduce the animal's activity and lead to boredom and obesity with resultant poor health, both physical and psychological. A balance therefore has to be struck between providing all that is required and making the animal work to acquire it. Some degree of physiological stress is necessary to achieve a well-balanced animal.

It is therefore necessary to consider the natural environment that the species in question has evolved to inhabit and then to consider how this can be reflected in the captive situation. For example, the Old World primate genus *Macaca* originated in Africa and then ultimately colonised much of southern and eastern Asia. There are 16–20 macaque species, which range as far north as 42°N in Japan to 9°S in Indonesia. Among the primates, only *Homo sapiens* exceeds the *Macaca* in the overall size of geographical range. The macaques are originally forest dwellers but many are very adaptable to different types of forest and non-forest habitats. They are found from sea level to altitudes up to 3000 m, in locations where snowfalls occur in winter to those where summer temperatures may be 50 °C, from dry desert areas to those with annual rainfall in excess of 100 cm, from deeply forested areas to highly urbanised environments with a close relationship with humans (Lindburg 1991). Some species such as *Macaca silenus* have very specific requirements (rainforest) whereas others such as *M. mulatta* are found across a whole range of habitat conditions. Knowledge of the macaques' ecological requirements is helpful in managing captive populations, whether for research or breeding. It will help to maximise breeding rates by improving birth rates and increasing reproductive lifespan.

While there may be similar trends present in many haplorhine species, the details will be different for some since they vary in their social relationships, use of space, level of activity and time and energy budgets, and in aspects of infant rearing, feeding and foraging.

Thus some practices when applied to a different species may have unforeseen and disastrous consequences and one should be aware of these potential pitfalls.

For example the behavioural and physiological differences between titi monkeys (*Callicebus moloch*) and squirrel monkeys (*Saimiri sciureus*) have a number of implications for their well-being (Mendoza 1991). These are both species of New World monkey and are very similar in size, cognitive capacity and nutritional requirements. However they differ markedly in their social interaction, their use of space and their response to change. The titi monkey is monogamous, lives in pairs and is territorial whereas the squirrel monkey lives in large multimale–multifemale groups roaming over a wide undefended area with no evidence of pair bonding (Terborgh 1983). The squirrel monkey is much bolder and more active than the titi and is less disrupted by the presence of strangers. These behavioural differences reflect underlying differences in their physiology; the squirrel monkey has a higher basal pituitary/adrenal activity and a higher heart rate (Mason 1991). This greater reactivity of the stress response does not imply that squirrel monkeys are more stressed than titi monkeys in comparable situations. The physiological response to stress does not of itself provide a measure of well-being, indeed the behavioural response indicates the reverse, that the titi monkeys are much more disrupted by altered conditions. Squirrel monkeys lead an active life and have physiological systems to promote energy use whereas in the titi monkey the physiological processes are designed for energy storage consistent with their more passive lifestyle. A large and varied environment is therefore more important to a squirrel monkey whereas predictable maintenance routines are important to the titi monkey. This physiological difference also reflects the type of clinical problem to which each species is more susceptible; the squirrel monkey, which has high sympathetic activity, is more susceptible to diseases such as atherosclerosis whereas the titi monkey is more prone to gastrointestinal disease reflecting the response to parasympathetic activity (Mason 1991). Making recommendations for maintaining captive species therefore requires knowledge of their behavioural responses, life history patterns and clinical tendencies.

There are currently many imperfections in the guidelines used to create housing for primates kept for research, and there are inconsistencies between regulations from different countries (Poole 1995). Sometimes space guidelines are incompatible with the recommendation that behavioural needs should be met and the wide discrepancies serve to throw doubt on the credibility of any of the recommendations. It is therefore important that these guidelines are under regular scrutiny and revision and that effort is made to have a unified approach that will best meet the needs of the animals.

Existing recommendations for primate housing, particularly in research facilities, are generally inadequate. Some are based solely on the weight of an animal without reference to linear dimensions. This can result in a cage which is actually smaller in the vertical dimension than the head to tail length of the monkey so that the animals cannot perch in the cage with the tail freely suspended, as they do in nature. The sizes of cages are sometimes too small to meet the behavioural needs of the animals; they provide neither adequate space for exercise nor room for environmental enrichment (see Figure 2.1). The assumption is made that heavier individuals require more space than lighter ones, although light, young animals are usually more active than the heavier adults. Use of engineering standards for the definition of cage dimensions will depend on such parameters as body weight, or

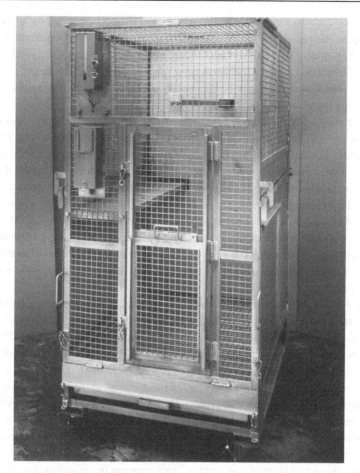

Figure 2.1   Conventional primate cage, within UK Home Office Code of Practice Guidelines but inadequate to provide for the animal's full behavioural needs.

dimension such as crown–rump length. It is better to use performance standards that assess the ability of the animal to express its species-typical behaviours, which will vary depending on species, age, sex, individual temperament, group composition and dynamics. It is important to appreciate that most recommendations for cage sizes represent *minimum* dimensions for animals of all ages. Duration of stay of the animal is also relevant. Where primates are to be kept for a period of years, the necessity for housing them in a better environment that satisfies their needs is even more important than for those animals that will only stay for a short while.

In healthy primate colonies it should not be necessary to clean and sterilise cage areas daily, to do so will remove the olfactory signals that are vital in the maintenance of the social hierarchy and the lack of these signals will cause disruption to the group. It is generally satisfactory simply to remove wet and soiled areas of substrate to reduce the incidence of disease hazard, and unpleasant odours. Cleaning of the cage or enclosure is then done at intervals using hot water with non-toxic detergent to remove organic material, followed by a clean-water rinse. However, where sterilisation is required by an experiment or to anticipate the possibility of an outbreak of disease, such as in a quarantine facility, animal holding areas can be designed so that, in the case of cages for small primates, they can be dismantled to place them in a cage wash or autoclave. For larger primates the whole room, including cages, may be cleaned by steam under pressure, and/or fumigated after relocating the primates elsewhere.

Cages are frequently constructed of metal with wire mesh walls, or parallel metal bars. This is not only expensive but cold to touch, noisy and not very animal friendly. It is easy to clean but this would not be highest on the animals' priority list if they could choose their own environment. Much preferred by the primates are materials that are warmer to the touch, chewable, able to be scent marked and provide a quieter environment than the clanking of metal cages. It is recommended that there is provision of some type of mesh or horizontal bars, to allow the animals to climb (MRC 2004). Wood may be used for cage construction and has the advantage of allowing greater adaptability in construction. Other materials such as Trespa can be used but these have the disadvantage of becoming quite slippery when wet, and are very heavy when used for removable partitions.

Individual cages are often made of stainless steel or aluminium with a squeeze back, which is a false back that can be drawn forward by the operator using handles on the front attached by poles or a pulley mechanism. The squeeze back is so named because it can be latched into position with the animal 'squeezed' right against the front of the cage, thus immobilising it, say, for an injection (see Figure 2.2). Most animals find this procedure very stressful and there are better ways to handle most monkeys (see Chapter 7).

The structural division of space in primate enclosures is of paramount importance. It is essential that the animals should be able to utilise as much of the volume as possible because, being arboreal, they occupy a three-dimensional space. To make this possible perches, swings and climbing structures should be provided. Visual barriers, which allow the animals to be out of sight of one another, are important in group housing and multiple escape routes provide opportunities to avoid attacks and also prevent dominant individuals from restricting access of subordinates to other parts of the cage. Where individuals need to be treated individually, as in toxicology experiments, areas with a partition to allow separation or social contact are required.

In a research setting a design that combines cages with an enclosure area is a flexible and useful solution to the conflict between wishing to give the animal free access to space and wishing to keep it in a cage to make it more accessible (see Figure 2.3). This permits the retention of a number of standard cages, allowing the animals to be removed into transport chairs for testing; but at the same time allowing them access to a much larger and more complex space when not working. In this setting the animals will show an extensive range of natural behaviours, little aggression and move quite readily into the transport chairs for testing. If the use of animals in research is to be supported there is an ethical obligation to house and maintain them in the best conditions that can be provided, so as 'best practice' evolves it is necessary to continually question if the facilities and their operation and management can be improved.

Bedding is not necessary as such, but a substrate such as shavings, hemp or sawdust should be provided in which food can be placed so the animals can forage for it,

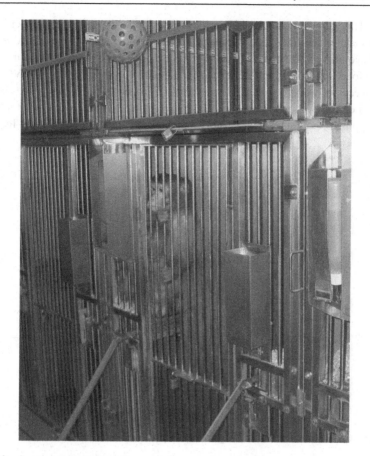

Figure 2.2   Squeeze back in operation.

which is a natural behaviour. Hay, straw or other material such as shredded paper may be provided for environmental enrichment. Marmosets benefit from and use nest boxes, preferably made of wood. Mesh floors allow the faeces to fall through and this may be a consideration for some procedures or in the presence of certain infectious diseases. However, primates that are ground dwellers rather than arboreal prefer a solid floor, where a layer of wood-chips, sawdust or bark chips will often be beneficial and allow foraging for food. The material must be non-toxic in case it is ingested with the food.

Environmental enrichment is essential for non-human primates to meet their ethological and psychological needs. It should provide the animals with the opportunity to carry out a sufficiently varied daily programme of activity. The actual enrichment provided will vary, but there is now a large literature offering a wide variety of options. Opportunities for the animals to exercise a full locomotory repertoire should be provided in the living area. To allow this, the cage must be sufficiently large and contain adequate furnishings. Cage furniture itself can provide opportunities for a wide repertoire of behaviour (see Figures 2.4a and 2.4b). Perches, ladders, swings, nets, toys to chew, plastic chains, car tyres etc. are all of value, and allow the animals plenty of places to sit without having to squabble. This allows the social hierarchy to develop with less aggressive encounters. Devices to encourage foraging (ranging from food scattered in the substrate to puzzle feeders) have proved effective (Figure 2.5). Some practical tips include the use of wire grids over food hoppers rather than expensive manufactured food puzzles, PVC perches or pipes, pieces of wood or branches, ice cubes of frozen juice, frozen grapes or melon cubes, food on top of the enclosure to encourage animals to forage upwards through the mesh, wrapping or boxing of treats, empty diet bags or cardboard boxes, gum feeders for

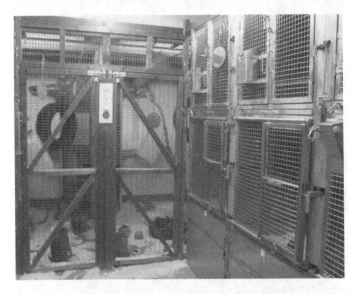

Figure 2.3   Combination of standard cages and an open enclosure.

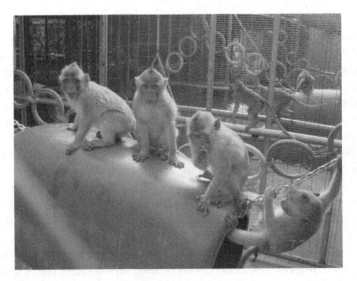

Figure 2.4a   Climbing enrichment (outdoors).

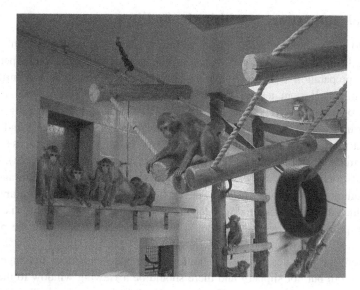

Figure 2.4b Climbing enrichment (indoors).

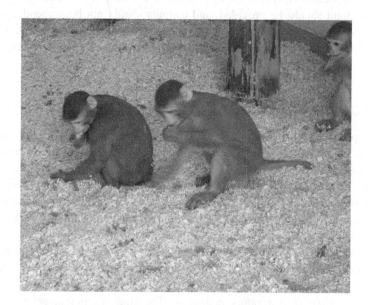

Figure 2.5 Foraging in substrate.

marmosets, and foraging boxes full of hay or sawdust (Heath & Libretto 1993; Dean 1999; Roberts *et al*. 1999). Novelty is important so the toys should be exchanged frequently. To avoid one animal monopolising a toy, more than one should be provided. Marmosets should be provided with wooden surfaces to gnaw, as this is part of their natural behaviour. Training animals to cooperate with carers and experimenters also helps to enrich the animal's life and reduces handling stress (Reinhardt & Reinhardt 2000) (see Chapter 7).

Functional support areas within the facility

In addition to animal holding areas, a primate facility should be equipped with many of the following facilities: secure delivery area, food storage areas, refrigeration for perishable food, a food preparation area, an equipment store for cage furnishings and enrichment apparatus, a treatment room, a surgical suite with operating room, preparation and support areas, a post-operative recovery area, nursery, specialist rooms for such investigations as radiology or ultrasound, isolation and quarantine areas with separate access and service areas, a post-mortem room with downdraft table or class 3 cabinet, carcase storage (fridge and freezer), storage for animal records (hard copy and/or electronic), shower facilities, staff rooms, office and administration areas, waste handling and storage areas, a clinical pathology laboratory, procedural areas with whatever special equipment is required. Which of these is required will depend on the purpose of the facility and the use to which the primates are put, but all should receive due consideration in the planning stages.

Areas where the primates are living should be equipped with floor drainage, floors should be smooth but not slippery and there should be a viewing window to the room. Walls should be protected against trolley damage by bumper guards, skirting should be coved, and lights and electrical fittings compatible with power washing. A daylight spectrum of light should be provided, and ceilings should not be suspended or allow access to ceiling voids in case of escape. Room should be monitored for both temperature and humidity, and each area should have access to a hose on a wall-mounted bracket and a squeegee.

INDOOR/OUTDOOR/COMBINATION FACILITIES?

Laboratory primates are often kept in cages or rooms, some larger species may be kept in outside pens or corrals, with free access to a heated indoor area. Many zoo primates are kept in a free-range parkland setting. There is a perception that there is a welfare advantage associated with the provision of external accommodation to all primates. However, it is the quality of the accommodation and the handling of the animals that matters most in terms of animal welfare and the mere fact of outdoor accommodation is not necessarily in itself a benefit.

External accommodation carries with it risks from exposure to wildlife (small birds, rodents, insects), disease transmission from outside vectors (e.g. *Mycobacteria, Salmonella, Yersinia*), or damage due to adverse climate conditions (e.g. frost injuries). These may predispose to enteric or respiratory pathology. The kind of external environment and what is provided within it, may be constrained by safety considerations for both animals and staff and by the practicalities of capture and of cost. Outside pens do not in any real way liberate the animals but simply offer access to a controlled external space. In human terms, open countryside, a garden and a prison yard are very different: each involves a different balance of risk and environmental quality. External runs offer access to outside air and a choice of environment, but will require measures to prevent escape of the monkeys and to ensure that wild animals are unable to gain entry; hence, the runs have grid or solid sides. Since the external enclosure for laboratory primates must not raise disease or safety risks it will typically have minimal vegetation and a concrete floor. If a 'parkland' setting, such as is often seen for zoo primates, were to become an option for laboratory primates, the animals would more realistically be classified as wild in origin, and this would restrict the legal and ethical decisions on the suitability for their use in research.

If the primates are kept outside, there should be shelter from adverse weather conditions, with at least a partial roof covering to provide protection from wind, rain and sun. The fabric of external enclosures and the materials used must be windproof and weatherproof, and of durable, impervious, cleanable materials. Since many primates choose to spend a substantial amount of their time foraging, anything that may restrict this should be regarded as potentially detrimental to their welfare, yet there may be limitations for providing deep litter for foraging since it could become soaked by rain or become a home for vermin and promote disease. In the laboratory setting where disease-free animals are required, these factors may reduce the supposed welfare gain of external accommodation over a good quality internal exercise area. A facility can be designed to maximise daylight by the incorporation of windows; and if the configuration of the building offers a choice between a place in a sunny/cool window region and a more controlled environment within the inner confines of the building this will allow the animals to select their own thermal environment.

The choice of internal accommodation will also facilitate animal handling and the desire to increase the extent to which the primates are accustomed to human contact and socialisation. Achieving this with a potentially aggressive species depends not only on staff education and training, but also on the configuration of the facilities, including plentiful enrichment, and accommodation that allows the animal refuge points from where it can interact with humans without feeling threatened. In the development of non-stressful and safe means of capture and in training animals, there should be dual emphasis on animal welfare and staff health and safety. These developments are only practicable in a building that allows for the seclusion of the occasional aggressive animal (sub-division of areas) for the protection of staff and other animals, and within which it is possible to train animals to come forward for capture and for simple interventions. Capture by means of netting (as is often used in large outside runs) is both stressful for the animals and a may be source of minor injuries. The stresses of handling for minor procedures can be greatly reduced by training, and monkeys are well able to learn to volunteer for these interventions (see Chapter 7).

The extent of the human–monkey interaction bears directly on intended end-use; familiarity with human handling is valuable in preparing animals for work in some studies. Initial profiling and training has potential benefits in selecting animals for different end-uses. This is more difficult to deliver without the kind of close contact that is possible in an internal facility. However for other types of study (such as studies of natural behaviour) it is necessary to have large naturalistic social groups (depending on the species) with diversity of demography and social and genetic relationships which are more achievable in a parkland type setting.

The final decision on whether to choose an internal, external or mixed facility will depend on factors including the use of the animals (laboratory, zoo, conservation, returning to the wild), the species, the local climate and cost. The facility must be 'fit for purpose' but there should be no underlying assumption that outside living areas are somehow automatically better. A well designed facility is vital in the delivery of a successful animal care programme and behavioural management (see Chapter 7). Building a new facility takes a long time from conception to completion and there will be many factors and details to consider. Cost, design, materials and utilities will inevitably be higher on the list of priorities for the build management team than species-specific behaviours of the animals to be housed in it.

ENVIRONMENTAL CONDITIONS

The environmental sensitivity of primates varies considerably from one species to another with some being more tolerant of environmental change than others. Some baboon species, e.g. hamadryas (*Papio hamadryas hamadryas*) and chacma (*P. h. ursinus*) flourish in semi- and sub-desert habitats, such as the Namib Desert (Namibia) where environmental temperatures may cause the core body temperature of baboons (*P. h. ursinus*) to reach as high as 42.7°C (Brain & Mitchell 1999). At the other extreme Japanese macaques (*Macaca fuscata*) occur at the highest latitude of any non-human primate, including in subalpine habitats (Rowe 1996). The most northerly populations of Japanese macaques grow a thick coat to cope with snowy conditions, some are even known to make use of hot springs to seek temporary respite from the cold.

In the wild, rhesus macaques (*M. mulatta*) occur across a wide range of altitudes from sea level to 3000 m (Rowe 1996) which indicates a tolerance of a substantial temperature range. Long-tailed macaques (*M. fascicularis*), on the other hand, may be less tolerant being found in habitat from sea level to 2000 m. The small New World species such as the common marmoset (*Callithrix jacchus*) inhabit a classic tropical forest habitat where seasonal changes are characterised more by variation in precipitation than in temperature. Most commonly the major changes in temperature in these habitats occur on a 24-hour cycle.

Although guidelines are published defining the environment in which primates should be housed, it is important that, as with all guidelines these should be viewed as the minimum requirements and those establishments wishing to demonstrate best practice should endeavour to produce conditions for their animals that exceed these in terms of their provision of a naturalistic environment. A naturalistic environment will contribute substantially to meeting a key recommendation of ethologists advising on the care and maintenance of captive primates: encouraging as natural a range and rate of behaviours as possible.

Temperature

The recommended temperature regimes for New and Old World primates relate to differences in the natural habitats to which they have adapted. In the UK a higher temperature range (20–28°C) is required for New World primates compared with that for Old World monkeys (15–24°C) and this reflects the difference between the exclusively tropical forest habitat of the former and the tropical to subtropical habitat of the latter (Wolfensohn & Lloyd 2003). In the USA the recommended temperature range is less specific being quoted as 18–24°C for all primates (NRC 1996). In this case the lower end of this range clearly falls outside that recommended in the UK for New World primates.

Depending on the location, and ambient temperature, of the facility housing primates these recommended temperatures will be achieved and maintained either through a system of heating or cooling. It is desirable that where heating/cooling is provided, temperature monitoring and thermostatic control is separate for each room. It should be borne in mind that stocking density will affect the temperature in each room, this would create significant temperature variation between rooms under a single heating/cooling system where stocking density varies significantly. As a contingency there should be an alternative power source (in case of power failure), also there should be enough capacity in the system to allow the powering of plant at lower than usual levels: to allow for running repair or maintenance. Sufficient fail-safe precautions should be built into the temperature control system to prevent potentially fatal temperature increases and ventilation failure in the event of plant failure.

While it remains undesirable for rapid fluctuations in temperature to exist in the housing, appropriate dampened temperature fluctuation on a 24-hour cycle that mimics natural temperature may help encourage natural behaviour such as taking a siesta during the hot part of the day and huddling at nights when it is cooler (Honess *et al.* 2004).

Where and when cooling is necessary, it should be remembered that air conditioning systems can result in a lowering of humidity (see below). Where animals are housed with outdoor access, a sufficiently cool interior should be available either in very hot northern, or southern, latitude summers or in hot climates. Where no interior housing is provided it is vital that sufficient shelter is available to allow the animals to shelter from climatic extremes (see below).

Ventilation

When animals are housed without outside access it is important that sufficient ventilation is provided. Under certain experimental regimes and containment levels it may be important to ensure negative air pressure in the animal rooms. In the UK 10 to 12 air changes per hour are required (Home Office Codes of Practice); 10 to 15 air changes per hour are recommended in the USA and recycled air should contain at least 50% fresh air (NRC 1996). It is important, however, to prevent drafts.

Where necessary, specialist advice should be sought on the use of a suitable system of air filtering, e.g. to prevent contamination with pathogens or to prevent the build-up of potentially damaging substances such as ammonia. Monitoring of filters is essential as dust from bedding, forage substrate or fur may block the filters or impair their function.

Relative humidity

Low humidity levels can result in skin problems and increased insensible fluid loss; while very high levels, although these may in some cases mimic humidity levels in the animal's natural environment, can result in thermoregulatory problems by prevention of evaporative cooling and can encourage the growth of fungi.

In the UK relative humidity levels are required to be 45–65% under the Home Office Code of Practice for the Housing & Care of Animals used in Scientific Procedures; and 40–70% under the Home Office Code of Practice for the Housing & Care of Animals in Designated Breeding and Supply Establishments. In the USA the recommended range is 30–70% for all primates (NRC 1996). As with temperature, it is desirable to have room-by-room monitoring and control of humidity levels. Efforts should be made to reduce the impact on conditions, such as humidity levels, of husbandry practices such as extensive cage/housing washing. Extensive daily washing, such as pressure-hosing may result in surfaces that remain permanently wet, resulting in elevated humidity levels and presenting a potential health risk to the animals as many pathogens remain viable in a warm, wet environment.

Protection from weather extremes

If an outside run is provided it is vital that the interior accommodation is sufficiently attractive that animals do not seek all their stimulation outside, particularly during periods of inclement weather.

To ensure that the most basic levels of welfare provision are met, it is vital that primates maintained outside in caging or corrals are afforded the opportunity to shelter from climatic extremes. The provision of shade from excessive and direct sun is essential, as is shelter from wind and heavy rain. Outside caging can be protected with natural vegetation or roofing over part or all of the length of the cage. During seasonally bad weather, sides and a ceiling can be attached to the caging for extra shelter and to allow heating of the interior. Where excessive heat may be a problem, this can be combated by providing a pool for recreational use and behavioural thermoregulation, or the thermo-statically controlled spraying of a fine mist of water droplets that can reduce the ambient temperature by in the region of 5°C (Honess *et al.* 2004).

Lighting

Where animals have access to daylight and are not maintained in a region where day lengths are the same as, or very similar to, those in the natural geographical range of the species it will be necessary to regulate lighting regimes. In most instances (except tropical breeding centres) the animals are held at higher latitudes than where the animals occur in the wild and therefore where day length is subject to greater variation. In northern latitudes it will be necessary to provide supplementary lighting during the winter months. Where access to daylight is not available a lighting regime of 12 hours light, 12 hours dark is typically provided, in which case efforts should be made to replicate dawn and dusk gradations in light intensity.

Special lighting provision is needed for captive primates. In the wild, primates rely on the ultraviolet in daylight to produce vitamin D_3. Care should be taken to ensure that, particularly in the absence of natural light, artificial light is provided using daylight spectrum tubes or bulbs rather than standard fluorescent lighting. While this is import-ant for both Old and New World primates, particularly the latter, it is also important where there may be a familial predisposition to metabolic bone disease or even, minor deficit in dietary vitamin D_3 (Wolfensohn 2003). Artificial lighting typically lacks a UV component and where this is the case or access to daylight limited, specific provision of UV light is recommended otherwise vitamin D_3 should be supplied as a supplement in the animals' diet (see Chapter 4).

Care should be taken in the positioning and intensity of artificial lighting in interior accommodation. Highly engineered caging such as that found in experimental facilities is frequently made of galvanised steel. Poorly positioned and overly intense lighting can intensify the glare from the often highly-polished metal surfaces. This can be reduced by using more sympathetic, better placed lighting and the use of brushed steel or better, more natural caging materials such as wood and wire (Figure 2.6).

The lighting system is also important in preventing the creation of overly dark parts of the caging, such as the lower levels or corners of shelved caging, in which potentially ill animals may hide from the eyes of monitoring animal care or veterinary staff.

Sound levels

The design of primate housing which seeks to ensure that it is both secure and easy to clean can mean that materials used for caging and the surfaces of the rooms, particularly in experimental facilities, do little to dampen any noise produced either by the animals or the staff going about their usual husbandry practices. High noise levels may intimidate many animals and have a negative effect on their psychological well-being.

There are four primary sources of noise: the primates themselves (e.g. vocalisations); the physical environment (e.g. caging, displaying, extractors, pumps); the staff (overshoes, shouting, husbandry, research, doors, capture); alarms, public address and entertainment systems (for staff and animals).

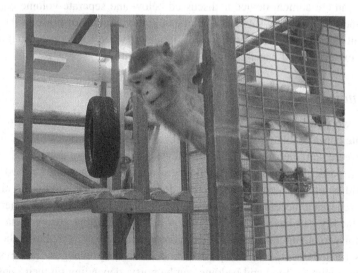

Figure 2.6   Use of wood and wire as enclosure materials.

Animal noise

Primates are highly social animals and one of their primary modes of communication is vocal. The noise, specifically the volume, produced through vocalisations varies between species and to an extent is related to body size. It is important that primates are permitted to communicate in this way both with conspecifics and animal care staff and in general vocal communication should be encouraged in captive primates. It should be borne in mind, however, that dominance can be asserted through vocalisations and therefore care needs to be taken in placement of overly assertive animals in proximity to those that may be negatively affected by vocal bullying.

Environment noise

The design of the physical environment and materials used in its construction can be responsible for substantial noise pollution. If cages are constructed using metal sheeting and heavy meshing with metal furniture, such as swings, then when larger primates display using their caging the noise production can be substantial. In fact even the dropping of toys, heavy food items or the tipping over of trays, pools etc. on a grid floor can be very noisy and can have a negative affect on nervous animals. Swings, particularly rigid metal ones, can also be used in displays of aggression, swung against the roof or sides of the cage creating intimidating noise and also presenting an injury risk to cage mates. The use of more natural caging construction and furnishing materials such as wood will help reduce noise, as will the provision of a solid, rather than a grid, floor covered with sound-dampening forage substrate such as wood chips.

Care needs to be taken over the placement of sirens for security, fire or system failure as well as speakers for public address, door alert or entertainment systems. Where possible sirens should not be sited too close to animal accommodation as these will undoubtedly cause extreme anxiety in the animals if any of the alarms should be triggered. The value of music as an enrichment device is discussed below and separate volume controls for corridors and animal rooms should be available. Other sources of noise in the physical environment that need to be taken into consideration when looking to minimise noise include air extractors and water pumps.

Human noise

The people who work around or with the primates, as well as those who visit the facility, can generate considerable noise. It may be reassuring for the animals to hear the voices of familiar care staff but not all staff are viewed as friendly by the animals and their voices may, particularly when loud, produce a response suggesting stress or anxiety. Staff should be encouraged to keep voices down and to work around the animals in a way that reduces unnecessary loud noises. Again, the materials and equipment used in a primate facility can have a strong affect on noise generation. Heavy metal modular caging is noisy to manipulate during cleaning, reorganisation or even during the catching of animals for treatment, research procedure or husbandry changes. Trolleys that are used to move animals, food and bedding can be noisy, depending on their construction, whether they frequently collide with corridor walls and doors and whether metal castors are used on hard floors. Other noise-generating factors such as slamming or banging doors, and clothing, including plastic overshoes, need to be considered when examining noise production and its prevention around captive primates.

Cleaning methods can also generate excessive noise: for example the use of high-pressure cleaning hoses on metal caging and pop-hole doors can produce anxiety in animals, even if they are excluded from the areas being cleaned. Managers will often require husbandry duties to be carried out to optimise the efficient use of staff time and as a result it is easy to overlook the effect their method of working has on the animals. Wherever possible husbandry duties should be carried out to minimise the impact on the animals being cared for, even if this is at the cost of working efficiency. Husbandry regimes that may be more labour-intensive but have a reduced impact on the animals should be used.

WASTE MANAGEMENT

Waste from a primate facility can be divided into animal carcases, clinical waste, animal waste including bedding materials, and office waste. The cleaning of cages and the disposal of animal waste is a specialised technique which needs to avoid the formation of aerosols of animal products in the environment. Such aerosols may settle only very slowly despite appropriate ventilation and may pose a hazard. Animal waste should be collected carefully, bagged in appropriate containers, labelled and disposed of according to national waste-disposal regulations. It must not be treated like household waste. Carcases and tissue specimens from animals may require double bagging in heavy gauge plastic bags of particular colour or labelling and should be collected for incineration by trained personnel. Included in clinical waste are needles and scalpels, which must be deposited carefully in a specialised sharps container and then taken to an authorised site by an authorised carrier. Office waste contains mainly paper, but may well contain material that is confidential, in which case it should be shredded inside the office before removal to the main waste container.

FURTHER RESEARCH NEEDED

While a good deal is known about the needs of non-human primates in captivity, there are a number of aspects where more scientifically validated information would be welcome to supplement the experience on which the present recommendations are largely based. Little is known of the effects of transportation on primates (Wolfensohn 1997). While it may seem ideal for primates to be bred in Europe, breeding in source countries has some advantages for the animals. These advantages, however, need to be balanced against any stress the animals may be subjected to as a result of the additional transportation. The increases in cage sizes and social housing recommended will make isolation of individuals less easy; more research is needed to develop improved techniques for handling and training primates. This will encourage the development of humane techniques to facilitate the movement of primates from one cage to another or to a particular area of the home cage.

FURTHER READING

Brain, C. & Mitchell, D. (1999) Body temperature changes in free-ranging baboons (*Papio hamadryas ursinus*) in the Namib Desert, Namibia. *International Journal of Primatology*, **20** (4), 585–598.

Dean, S.W. (1999) Environmental enrichment of laboratory animals used in regulatory toxicology studies. *Laboratory Animals*, **33**, 309–327.

Fortman, J.D., Hewett, T.A. & Taylor Bennett, B. (2002) *The Laboratory Non-human Primate*. CRC Press, Boca Raton, Florida.

Heath, M. & Libretto, S.E. (1993) Environmental enrichment for large-scale marmoset units. *Animal Technology*, **44**, 163–173.

The Home Office Code of Practice for the Housing and Care of Animals used in Scientific Procedures. HMSO, London.

The Home Office Code of Practice for the Housing and Care of Animals in Designated Breeding and Supplying Establishments. HMSO, London.

Honess, P., Johnson, P. & Wolfensohn, S. (2004) A study of behavioural responses of non-human primates to air transport and re-housing. *Laboratory Animals*, **38**, 119–132.

IPS (1993) International Guidelines for the acquisition, care and breeding of non-human primates. *Primate Report*, Special Issue. International Primatological Society. Erlick Goltze, Göttingen, Germany.

Karl, J. & Rothe, H. (1996) Influence of cage size and cage equipment on physiology and behaviour of common marmosets. *Laboratory Primate Newsletter*, **35**, 10–14.

Lindburg, D.G. (1991) Ecological requirements of macaques. *Laboratory Animal Science*, **41**, 315–322.

Mason, W.A. (1991) Effects of social interaction on well-being: developmental aspects. *Laboratory Animal Science*, **41**, 323–328

Mendoza, S.P. (1991) Sociophysiology of well-being in non-human primates. *Laboratory Animal Science*, **41**, 344–349.

MRC (2004) *MRC Ethics Guide: Best Practice in the Accommodation and Care of Primates used in Scientific Procedures*. Medical Research Council, London.

Napier, J.R. & Napier, P.H. (1985) *The Natural History of the Non-Human Primates*. Cambridge University Press, Cambridge.

NRC (1996) *Guide for the Care and Use of Laboratory Animals*. National Research Council. National Academy Press, Washington D.C.

NRC (1997) *The Psychological Well-Being of Non-Human Primates*. National Research Council. National Academy Press, Washington D.C.

Poole, T. (1995) Guidelines and legal codes for the welfare of non-human primates in biomedical research. *Laboratory Animals*, **29**, 244–249.

Poole, T.B. (ed.) (1999) *The UFAW Handbook on the Care and Management of Laboratory Animals*, 7th edn. Blackwell Science, Oxford.

Reinhardt, V. & Reinhardt, A. (2000) Social enhancement for adult non-human primates in research laboratories. *Laboratory Animals*, **29**, 34–41.

Reinhardt, V. & Reinhardt, A. (2002) *Comfortable Quarters for Laboratory Animals*, 9th edn. Animal Welfare Institute, Washington D.C.

Reinhardt, V. & Seelig, D. (1998) *Environmental Enhancement for Caged Rhesus Macaques: A Photographic Documentation*. Animal Welfare Institute, Washington D.C.

Roberts, R.L., Roytburd, L.A. & Newman, J.D. (1999) Puzzle feeders and gum feeders as environmental enrichment for common marmosets. *Contemporary Topics in Laboratory Animal Science*, **38**, 27–31.

Röder, E.L. & Timmermans, P.J.A. (2002) Housing and care of monkeys and apes in laboratories: adaptations allowing essential species-specific behaviour. *Laboratory Animals*, **36**, 221–242.

Rowe, N. (1996) *A Pictorial Guide to the Living Primates*. Pogonias Press, East Hampton, New York.

Taylor Bennett, B., Abee, C.R. & Henrickson, R. (eds) (1995) *Non-human Primates in Biomedical Research: Biology and Management*. American College of Laboratory Animal Medicine Series. Academic Press, New York.

Terborgh, J. (1983) *Five New World Primates: A Study in Comparative Ecology*. Princeton University Press, Princeton, New Jersey.

Wolfensohn, S.E. (1993) The use of microchip implants in identification of two species of macaque. *Animal Welfare*, **2**, 353–359

Wolfensohn, S.E. (1997) Brief review of scientific studies of the welfare implications of transporting primates. *Laboratory Animals*, **31**, 303–305.

Wolfensohn, S.E. (2003) Case report of a possible familial predisposition to metabolic bone disease in juvenile rhesus macaques. *Laboratory Animals*, **37**, 139–144.

Wolfensohn, S.E. & Lloyd, M.H. (2003) *Handbook of Laboratory Animal Management and Welfare*, 3rd edn. Blackwell Science, Oxford.

Chapter 3
Staff management and health and safety

SELECTION OF STAFF

Animal facilities do not run themselves and the care that the animals receive depends totally on the staff who provide it. Recruitment and selection of skilled, motivated and empathetic staff are essential to a good animal care programme. Working with primates is a very rewarding career at all levels and provides many opportunities for fulfilment. No matter what experience staff arrive with, they will require on-going training and development if they are to maximise their potential.

TRAINING OF STAFF

A good training programme will assist in staff retention, reduce turnover and benefit the animals. The aims of the training programme should include the following elements:

- a greater understanding of primate ethology and biology (Chapter 1);
- an overview of the organisations associated with primate use and its governance (Chapter 1);
- a broader understanding of the issues of use and supply of primates (Chapter 1);
- an understanding of safety issues (this chapter);
- the knowledge and tools to make refinements in the management of primates (Chapters 2, 4, 5 and 6);
- a mechanism for evaluating primate welfare through behavioural indices (Chapters 6 and 7).

There are many individuals, such as care, veterinary, and research staff, as well as students, and ethical committee members, who make up the multi-disciplinary teams that are associated with primate care in the various types of institution. Obtaining agreement on the importance of staff training is straightforward, but getting implementation and participation of the team members, who will have a wide diversity of education and experience, can be more of a challenge.

HEALTH AND SAFETY ISSUES

When employing staff to work with primates, there are a number of specific considerations in relation to the health and safety aspects of such work, which need to be addressed. Within the European Community, a number of Directives under the Treaty of Rome's Article 118A relate to health and safety and have been adopted by member states. The Framework Directive sets out general principles for employers to follow. The Workplace Directive contains minimum health, safety and welfare requirements for permanent workplaces. The Use of Personal Protective Equipment Directive deals with the selection and maintenance of suitable protective clothing and other equipment.

Occupational health and safety personnel will need a detailed knowledge of legislation in order to be able to translate it into working practices. In many countries, some occupational diseases such as occupational asthma and some zoonoses must be reported to government agencies, and compensation may be awarded to personnel developing such 'prescribed' occupational diseases. Employers are required to respond to employee risk factors, and may have to make difficult decisions about suitability for work both before and during employment. If appropriate action to protect employees is not taken, then the enforcement authorities may well resort to legal action against the employer. Increasingly, insurance companies are requiring details of potential hazards and risks in the workplace, and evidence of suitable methods of control, before they will issue policies to employers.

The field of occupational health and safety is a constantly changing one. The emergence of new hazards presents challenges to employers who must protect their employees; the emergence of new methods of working with animals presents challenges to users who must improve animal welfare. It is incumbent on those who are responsible for primate facilities to develop, improve and implement a programme that is an appropriate balance of the two.

The Occupational Health and Safety Programme

Surveys have shown that any animal care occupation has a wide variety of work-place hazards, they are not unique to non-human primates (ACDP 1997, http://www.hsebooks. com). All potential hazards should be identified and then appropriate steps taken to reduce the risks. The Occupational Health and Safety Programme (OHSP) should identify the hazards, determine the risks associated with them, design a management programme to reduce the risks and communicate all these hazards, risks and safety measures to the employees. The OHSP should promote a culture of safety in the workplace. The cornerstone of a successful OHSP is strong administrative support. The OHSP team should include staff from the following groups: animal care, veterinary, research, environmental health and safety, occupational health and safety, administration and management with previous OHS experience.

Hazards associated with non-human primates

Since non-human primates and humans have a very close phylogenetic relationship, there are a number of pathogenic organisms that can be transmitted from them to humans and *vice versa*. The risk of transmission may potentially be greater than if working with many other animal species. It is therefore important to identify any possible hazards that the monkey may be carrying in order to be able to take steps to reduce the likelihood of any potential exposure. Health screening of the animals is a very important part of the OHSP in identifying such hazards. Pathogens may be transmitted to humans by a variety of routes including bites, scratches, needle-stick injuries, aerosol, splashing on to mucous membranes or by accidental ingestion. Once the hazard has been identified control measures must look at the possible routes of transmission for that organism. Some infectious agents may not cause overt disease in the monkey but may be carried subclinically, these organisms must still be identified and adequate steps taken to prevent transmission. There are a number of potential pathogens and their relative significance will vary depending on the species of primate and the biology and epidemiology of the agents. This information is constantly being reviewed as our knowledge expands and the OHSP must also be reviewed regularly to take account of new information as it comes to light. An evaluation is required that considers the existing state of knowledge, any history of previous incidents and the likelihood of accidental exposure. This is less for agents that require intermediate hosts such as arthropod vectors. For primates used in research the OHSP must also take into account any infectious agents that are experimentally induced in the animals or that may be transmitted during xenotransplantation.

Viruses

B virus

The most significant potential zoonotic infection is probably B virus (*Herpesvirus simiae*). This virus occurs in Old World monkeys (but not apes) and has caused at least 40 cases of disease in humans, many of which were fatal (Holmes *et al.* 1995). Some human cases have occurred despite only minimal exposure to animals when wearing appropriate protective clothing. Considering the number of macaques that have been used in research, human cases are very rare; but the hazard still remains high although the risk is low. Control methods for research monkeys include only using animals from populations that are regularly screened for the disease and where all are found to be negative. Different serological tests vary in their sensitivity and specificity, so care should be taken when interpreting single results (see Chapter 5). Avoidance of bites and spitting, by careful handling and welfare techniques, is also required, combined with barrier methods of protection where appropriate.

Simian retroviruses

These are a complex group of related viruses including simian retrovirus type D and simian T-lymphotropic virus. Simian immunodeficiency virus (a lentivirus) can cause an AIDS-like syndrome in monkeys and there are a small number of case reports of transmission to humans through accidental exposure, but as yet none of the individuals has suffered clinical disease, although they demonstrate seroconversion. Simian foamy virus is also capable of transmission to humans but there is no evidence of pathogenicity in either humans or non-human primates (Centers for Disease Control 1997).

Other viruses to consider

Filoviruses (e.g. Marburg, Ebola), poxviruses, flaviviruses (e.g. yellow fever and dengue), lymphocytic choriomenigitis virus, rabies virus, simian virus 40 (SV-40), hepatitis A and hepatitis B should all be considered.

Bacterial disease

Tuberculosis, *Shigella*, *Salmonella*, *Campylobacter*, meliodosis, leprosy, and infections from bite wounds should be considered.

Protozoa

Entamoeba, *Balantidium*, *Cryptosporidium*, *Giardia*, malaria, *Toxoplasma*, trypanosomes, *Hymenolepsis*, *Oesophagostomum*, oxyurids, *Strongyloides* and *Trichuris* may be present.

For further details on infectious diseases of primates see Chapter 5.
    There may also be risks associated with use of invertebrates included in food.

Non-infectious hazards

Non-infectious hazards will include trauma from animal bites and scratches (Zakaria *et al.*, 1996). One solution is to prevent bites and scratches by working at a distance from the animal so that it never has the opportunity to make contact with the member of staff. This can be done by the application of engineering controls and use of such devices as crush backs and tunnel catching systems. Chemical control such as the tranquilisation of the animal before handling will also reduce the risks. However with both of these there is still a risk that an animal will grab at staff causing scratch injuries and there will be no trust between animal and carer. The use of personal protective equipment (PPE) such as Kevlar® gloves will reduce injuries. The alternative way to reduce the risk of injuries from the animal is to train it, using positive reinforcement techniques, to cooperate with routine husbandry procedures and to develop a culture in which the staff understand and anticipate primate behaviour and the primate expresses a normal repertoire of such behaviour (see Chapter 7).

Risk assessment

Risk assessment is the basis for designing and managing OHSPs to reduce workplace risks to an acceptable level. Zero risk is, for most activities, an unrealistic objective; so there is already an opportunity for divergent views on what constitutes an 'acceptable' level. The first step in risk assessment is hazard identification. Once hazards have been identified, the risks associated with them are identified and this process is known as risk assessment. The risk assessment is a tool that provides a rational framework within which to design and manage the OHSP. Its purpose is to determine the probability of injury or illness due to specific hazards, and this then becomes the basis of risk management through the OHSP. It enables the rational definition of safe working practices to protect employees, provides targets for managers for injury prevention, sets workplace standards and monitors compliance for regulators.

The hazards may be biological (e.g. infectious disease), chemical (e.g. disinfectants) or physical (e.g. slippery floors). Hazard identification must also include knowledge of the biology and behaviour of the primate species in question since experience of working with one species cannot necessarily be translated to working with another, and may therefore affect the level of risk involved.

All staff working with non-human primates should receive training in understanding primate behaviour (see Chapter 6 and 7), since this will assist in predicting their actions and thus reduce the risk of injury. It is necessary to understand primate facial expressions and body language; and the different interpretation of facial signals (Bayne *et al.* 1993). Any interaction needs to be based on a full understanding of the audio and visual cues specific to that primate species and staff training is these areas is vital. Good background knowledge will assist with predicting an animal's behaviour and thus identifying potential hazards, and added to this should be more detailed knowledge about the individual animal. This training should form part of the staff continuing professional development programme. The risk of injury can further be reduced by training the animals to cooperate in specific activities such as cage cleaning. A well-designed behavioural management programme can be a useful tool for reducing the risks associated with working with non-human primates. However each component of a behavioural management programme also poses its own challenges in the OHSP. Animals that exhibit behavioural pathology resulting from inadequate captive conditions can be unpredictable and aggressive and will thus present a hazard and high level of risk to workers. If animals are maintained in a state of well-being so they express more species-typical behaviour they will be more predictable and worker safety will improve. If the animals also associate the presence of such workers with positive experiences such as food treats or cognitive activities, they will be affiliative rather then aggressive toward the staff and their tendency will be such as to cooperate in the activity. Care must be taken that the animals do not form social hierarchies that inadvertently involve the staff through acts of aggression or submission. This will also protect staff safety.

The SOP (standard operating procedure) is central to safeguarding those at risk. The SOP will specify procedures that will maximise animal welfare but will also minimise potential risk to the individual. They are customised to the facility (e.g. research unit, zoo, breeding centre) and the different categories of people therein (care staff, veterinary staff, visitors, students) who will be engaged in different activities with the animals at varying degrees of proximity. There should be training programmes available for each category of worker so that they can receive the necessary information on potential hazards and avoidance of risks.

Assessment of risk will depend on an evaluation of hazards posed by the animals and/or by materials used with the animals. Identification of hazards will depend on observation, experience, published reports and professional judgement. Hazards typically found in primate units may be listed as follows:

1. *Needle stick, sharps injuries.* The use of engineering controls to ensure safe disposal of sharps and good staff training is essential in preventing this.
2. *Slips, trips and falls.* All animal facilities carry the risk of slips on wet floors, in primate units there may be bulky items of environmental enrichment equipment lying

around which can be a hazard. Staff training and having adequate space in which to work is essential, as well as utilising non-slip surfaces.

3. *Muscle strain*. Repetitive strain injury and muscular over-exertion are risks when dealing with large heavy items of equipment such as forage trays or wooden items of environmental enrichment. Good ergonomic design, adequate space and use of lifting equipment combined with staff training are essential.
4. *Burns*. These are possible from steam and pressure washers and autoclaves.
5. *Noise*. Noise levels can be high around cage washers, when cages or equipment are moved or when using mechanical equipment.
6. *Allergies*. These may develop to protective latex gloves or animal bedding products.
7. *Heat stress*. This can occur from use of PPE as it can get very hot in an all-in-one coverall suit when washing down primate areas. PPE goggles can steam up and reduce visual acuity which may then increase the risks.
8. *Chemical hazards*. Such things as disinfectants, volatile anaesthetics and injectable drugs may cause irritation of skin and mucous membranes, including the respiratory tract and/or sensitisation of the skin and lungs. Appropriate handling techniques are described by the manufacturers and should be available.

Risk assessment will take into account exposure intensity and frequency. Once the hazard has been identified and the necessary dose to cause harm has been determined, then the exposure is assessed, which will require evaluation of individual workers' skills, experience, job duties and the use of PPE.

1. *Individual susceptibility of the employee* may vary, for example, if immunosuppressed or pregnant, and will affect the risk assessment. Exposure control will depend on a combination of engineering controls, work practices and PPE to enable safe operating practices.
2. *Engineering controls* relate to use of air flows, filters, double-access door barriers, cage design, use of crush backs and catching tunnels and covers on electrical outlets where water is in use.
3. *Work practices* depend on adequate employee training. The first element of safe working practice is personal hygiene and primate workers should be provided with dedicated work clothing that is left at the facility. Frequent, regular and thorough hand washing should be encouraged and use of modern hand-cleansing units will reduce the incidence of any associated dermatitis. Encouragement of good housekeeping, with the promotion of a clean and uncluttered workplace, will reduce the potential for slips, trips and injuries. Staff training and experience is essential in the safe handling of animals. Any human–animal interaction depends on a thorough knowledge of the primate species and understanding of its behaviour and of the individual animal's own disposition, if the encounter is to be managed in a way that reduces the risk of injury. Use of low-pressure hoses will reduce aerosol formation and help reduce the exposure to some pathogens; dry cleaning and removal of waste should be managed in a way that minimises ergonomic stress and optimises infection control and animal welfare.

The risk to workers, on which the risk assessment is based, may be estimated by the expected incidence rate, which is represented by the following formula (NRC 2003):

$$\text{The incidence rate } = \frac{\text{Frequency of the event (or number of new occurrences)}}{\text{Average number of people at risk for the event}}$$

It is important to understand that there is an inherent uncertainty in risk assessment, but that reducing that uncertainty does not necessarily reduce (or increase) the risk. There are often limited data for quantifying risk factors which, combined with inherent variability and different information sources will contribute to uncertainties in estimates of risk. Any history of incidents is important in making the assessment by referring back to illness and injury in the facility's experience, near-miss reports and to reference material. Regulatory requirements may dictate the response to some levels of risk assessment.

Once the risk assessment has been completed, a course of action is formulated and implemented to mitigate the hazards. This is known as risk management. Hazards can be managed by various adjustments in work practice, equipment and facilities. Sometimes modifications will depend on engineering controls (facilities and equipment), sometimes on administrative changes (such as changes in the delegation of decision-making authority), changes in methodology and work practices (for example by training the animals) or adoption of new protective equipment.

Personal protective equipment (PPE)

Some form of PPE is essential when working with primates. The determination of the appropriate PPE will depend on the primate species, the health status of the animals and the people, and the work environment; but as a minimum will consist of dedicated workplace clothing and footwear. Workers must be trained in the appropriate selection, fitting and use of any other additions, which may include gloves, mask, hat, goggles and/or face visors. The use of such PPE may impede non-verbal communication with the primates and may actually increase risk during interaction between animal and staff. It is well recognised that new employees and those with less than 2 years' experience of working with primates are at a higher risk of injury. Decisions about the training and supervision of such staff and the types of PPE they should wear as well as the types of work they can carry out should be part of the risk management plan.

Review of Occupational Health and Safety Programme

Whatever the size of the facility there must be adequate resources for developing, managing and reviewing the institution's OHSP. There must be a specialised staff-training programme, which must consider the specific species of primate to be used since these vary widely in size and source, and will therefore affect the hazards to which staff may be exposed. The institute must make a commitment to the associated costs of an occupational health professional, employee screening (for example, for freedom from tuberculosis), vaccinations etc. as required. Employees should have ready access to hand-washing facilities and showers, eye-wash stations and emergency kits. Locker rooms and staff rest areas should be designed to minimise cross-contamination between these areas and animal areas.

It is necessary to have a plan for information management and regular review of the OHSP, injury log and a retraining plan if necessary.

Every unit should also have an emergency plan for dealing with disasters including fires, power failures, earthquakes, flood or other emergency such as attacks on property or personnel. There should be a specific plan for animal escape which will minimise employee hazards and risks. The emergency action plan should identify the responsibilities of personnel and provide readily accessible contact numbers for additional expertise and resources.

The OHSP should be evaluated regularly; if the unit is part of a larger organisation it is useful to involve the institutional occupational health and safety staff in this review, as this will provide a new perspective on programme design and implementation and will complement the perspective of the facility manger and senior staff.

Many factors will influence risk management: politics, economics, legal issues and technical concerns will affect the process, both locally and nationally. Sometimes financial constraints will lead to less than optimal risk-management decisions, and sometimes external influences will force over-conservative risk-management decisions. There must be a specific OHS plan and an appropriate safety culture and working environment. This will reflect the way that the institutional management and the staff feel about risk and how the organisation will tolerate risk in its daily activities. This attitude may differ between institutions.

Staff training

To maintain a safe working environment there must be a commitment to staff training, and, as there is dependence on safe working practices, staff must be aware of these practices, must be kept up to date and not allowed to drift back to older methods. A continual programme of training must be in place to take account of staff turnover and the development of working practices. Employees must know the hazards and understand how these are controlled through work practices, engineering controls and PPE. An effective training programme requires resources, administrative support, record keeping and a system for monitoring the training efficacy. It should be delivered routinely, not just when an incident occurs. There should be review of past performance, illness and injury reports, absentee records and staff concerns about safety and health; and an assessment to identify discrepancies between what people are actually doing, and the prescribed way to do it safely. Training objectives should reflect the desired training outcomes. The objectives break down into performance (the task to be done), condition (under which it is done) and criteria (the performance being measured and the standards against which it is measured) and they should be Specific, Measurable, Attainable, Relevant and in a given Timeframe (SMART). The content of training should be what the trainee must know rather than what he should or could know. Topics presented in training should include facility orientation, facility safety programme, hazards, PPE, first aid, material safety data sheets, SOPs, species-specific behaviour, sharps safety, protection of the back and the safe movement of equipment. It is necessary to have a programme of continuing education and to keep records of the outcomes.

LONE WORKING

In some occupations there are identified hazards and particular risks in working alone. This is especially so for animal handlers, particularly out in the field, with the possibility of severe injury. In all cases workers must have a rapid means of communication to someone who can respond on their behalf. This is naturally much easier in a purpose-built facility in the middle of a centre of population, but may be impracticable in certain remote locations. Such workers accept the (theoretically) greater risks associated with such work, but in order to make this judgement they must be aware of the potential risks and make their own assessment in conjunction with their employer. Some lone workers carry alarms which are activated if they change position rapidly, and in certain areas carrying personal radios or portable telephones is an option which should be considered. Workers should be sure that somebody knows where they are and must not deviate from their plans without informing a responsible person, however tempting an alternative scenario may be. Checking into and out of animal facilities with security coded entrances is now common and an added reassurance for the lone worker.

EMPLOYEE SECURITY

The very real problem associated with animal rights groups worldwide poses a considerable threat to the personal security of primate handlers in laboratory facilities. Primate facilities should be especially secure and will require high levels of entrance/exit control. The building should be designed so that breaking and entering is difficult or impossible and high levels of alarm systems connected to local police facilities are indicated.

Individual employees of such institutes may wish their identity to remain confidential. In particular the home addresses and telephone numbers of primate handlers should be kept completely confidential in secure storage. Such employees should not carry identification which indicates that they are primate handlers unless absolutely necessary.

However, it is advised that primate handlers should carry a card indicating the nature of their work in general terms. This should increase the 'index of suspicion' of a doctor or health facility to whom they are unknown, if they are taken ill perhaps in a remote or strange location. This 'hazcard' should be worded carefully and should not identify the individual's address, telephone number or next of kin.

FURTHER READING

ACDP (1997) *Working Safely with Research Animals: Management of Infection Risks.* Advisory Committee on Dangerous Pathogens. The Stationery Office, London.

Bayne, K.A.L., Dexter, S.L. & Strange, G.M. (1993) The effects of food treat provisioning and human interaction on the behavioural well-being of rhesus monkeys (*Macaca mulatta*). *Contemporary Topics in Laboratory Animal Science*, **32**, 6–9.

Centers for Disease Control and Prevention (1997) Non-human primate spumavirus infections among persons with occupational exposure. *Morbidity and Mortality Weekly Report*, **46**, 6.

Health and Safety Commission (1992) *Health and Safety in Animal Facilities*. Education Services Advisory Committee. HMSO, London.

Health and Safety Commission (1993) *Control of Substances Hazardous to Health.* General Approved Code of Practice, 4th edn. HMSO, London.

Holland, C. (ed.) (1997) *Modern Perspectives on Zoonoses.* Royal Irish Academy, Dublin.

Holmes, G.P., Chapman, L.E., Stewart, J.A., *et al.,* and the B virus working group (1995) Guidelines for the prevention and treatment of B-virus infections in exposed persons. *Clinical Infectious Diseases,* **20**, 421–49.

ILAR (1997) *Occupational Health and Safety in the Care and Use of Research Animals.* Institute of Laboratory Animal Resources. National Academy Press, Washington, D.C.

ILAR News (2003) Issue on: Occupational Health and Safety in Biomedical Research. Institute of Laboratory Animal Resources, **44** (1).

MRC (1990) *The Management of Simians in Relation to Infectious Hazards to Staff.* Medical Research Council Simian Virus Committee, London.

NRC (2003) *Occupational Health and Safety in the Care and Use of Nonhuman Primates.* National Research Council of the National Academies. National Academy Press, Washington D.C.

Zakaria, M., Lerche, N.W., Chomel, B.B. & Kass, P.H. (1996) Accidental injuries associated with nonhuman primate exposure at two regional primate research centres (USA) 1988–1993. *Laboratory Animal Science,* **46**, 298–304.

Chapter 4
Nutrition

NATURAL FEEDING ECOLOGY

In the wild state, the gathering of food is the principal activity for primates, and yet it is the most profoundly affected activity of a captive existence. Analysis of activity budgets in the wild has shown that more time is given to this activity than to any other (Lindburg 1991). Free-ranging primates spend a lot of time collecting and eating food, not just to satisfy their physiological needs but also because this is important in the behavioural and social life of primates. In captivity, providing food removes the need to forage to survive, and food tends to be presented to a predictable schedule. It is better to provide small portions less predictably to satisfy the animal's behavioural needs than to provide large portions primarily to satisfy the energy requirements.

Primate diets may, in crude terms, be classified as either faunivorous (animal-eating, including insect-eating), gummivorous (gum-eating), frugivorous (fruit-eating) or folivorous (leaf-eating) depending on the principal component of the diet. While this classification implies exclusivity, in reality primate diets are complex, including a mix of food types. While most species whether primarily folivorous, gummivorous or faunivorous include some fruit in their diet, none combines large proportions of leaf and insect food (Martin 1990). It is also possible to subdivide each diet type, for example the term 'faunivorous' includes both those that eat insects (insectivorous) and those that eat meat (carnivorous). Only the tarsiers (*Tarsius* spp.) among primates eat nothing but faunivorous diets and most primates are primarily plant eaters. Different species eat different parts of the plant, with folivores preferring mature leaves, young leaves, shoots or other plant parts, and frugivores selecting from the fruit pulp, seeds and skin. Both may eat flowers and buds. In some species certain parts are digested, whereas in others, if these are eaten, they may pass out in the faeces.

For all primates the feeding time makes up a significant percentage of all the daily activities, but for insectivores the time spent foraging for, capturing and eating the insects may be disproportionately high for the percentage of dietary intake and nutrition provided. Gummivores may rely on a very few species of trees. It is therefore necessary to consider in the feeding time both the forage time and the eating time. Food intake cannot be measured adequately by simply referring to the grams of food taken (how much fruit?). It is necessary to consider how much is consumed, how much is wasted, which part is consumed (and the nutrient content of that part) and whether or not that part is digested. The weight of the food may be misleading since fruit has a very high water content and it is therefore necessary to consider the percentage dry matter (%DM) of different foods in order for them to be compared. However the fibre component may be indigestible and for these foods although the %DM may be high, they are not very nutritious. It is therefore necessary to consider the metabolisable energy value and the nutrient content of the food but this can be difficult to obtain. There are very useful tables of nutrient content in foods commonly used to feed primates in *Nutrient Requirements of Non-human Primates* published by the National Research Council (NRC 2003a).

Omnivores are much more adaptable and so it is much easier to keep these species in captivity. Macaques consume principally wild fruits although they are flexible in their dietary preferences consuming a variety of plant and animal matter. However the components of the diet come in small aliquots, dispersed over a wide area (e.g. seeds, buds, flowers), so the process of gathering them is very time consuming and demands much energy. The macaque has to travel from area to area to find sufficient food and must compete in each area for the limited quantities that are available at each location. The daily activity cycle reflects this need as each day a troop of macaques will move to the first feeding site and spend the morning foraging, spreading out over the area as it does so. There is a siesta period in the middle of the day, then another bout of food gathering through the afternoon while progressing to the sleeping site, then grooming and sleep. The hands, feet, teeth, jaws and cheek pouches are all used for the gathering and processing of the small food components of the diet, adding interest and variety to the task of feeding.

In the wild there will be seasonal extremes, so the food eaten may depend on availability and necessity rather than on preference. The diet of captive primates needs to match the gastrointestinal (GI) system of the species for there is wide diversity across the order Primates. To create a suitable diet for a primate it is necessary to consider:

- foraging and feeding behaviour
- the structure and function of the digestive system
- the options and constraints imposed by captive dietary husbandry.

Each species has evolved to exploit specific food types and this is reflected in the structure of their dentition and gut morphology (Fleagle 1999). Primates are unusual among mammals in the diverse digestive tract structures found in the stomach, caecum and colon (Chivers & Hladik 1980). Faunivores (such as the angwantibo *Arctocebus calabarensis*) have a simpler and shorter GI tract than folivores. Cercopithecine primates (except the colobines) have cheek pouches into which harvested food can be stored short term. Primates, including those that are *primarily* frugivorous, have adopted two different strategies in order to deal with leafy dietary components containing cellulose, which primates cannot digest. The cellulose is instead fermented by symbiotic bacteria with the host absorbing the products of this process. Different species may be termed either foregut or hindgut fermenters. In the former the bacteria are housed in special compartments of an enlarged stomach (e.g. colobine monkeys) and in the latter they are housed in an enlarged caecum (e.g. sportive lemurs, *Lepilemur* spp.) or colon (e.g. howler monkeys, *Alouatta* spp., and some cercopithecine monkeys such as rhesus macaques, *Macaca mulatta* and vervet monkeys, *Cercopithecus aethiops*) (Fleagle 1999). Areas of the gut where fermenting takes place may also play a role in neutralising the effect of various toxic plant substances.

DIET FORMULATION AND PROCESSING

In closed-formula diets the specific amount of each ingredient is not revealed but there are estimates of typical nutrient content. Some feed formulations vary routinely depending on the quality and availability of feed ingredients; there may therefore be changes in some dietary constituents, such as phytoestrogens, which may have a significant impact, for example on reproductive efficiency or tumour growth. It is therefore better to use fixed-formula diets where the amount and identity of each ingredient is defined – but these diets are usually more expensive.

Primate diets are usually prepared by extrusion (expansion) or pelleting. In extrusion, the finely ground feed ingredients are subjected to high temperature (produced by injection of steam and mechanical friction) and high pressure. The temperature rises to about 130–150°C in the extruder barrel. These conditions are much more severe than seen in pelleting and lead to greater cooking of carbohydrates. Extruded diets are usually easier to eat, and more palatable and digestible than pelleted diets. Both the extruding and the pelleting processes will destroy some of the vitamins, especially vitamins A, D, E, C, thiamine and folic acid. Storage of diets in unsuitable conditions will also lead to a loss of vitamin content but in cool and dry conditions the level should remain adequate for several months. Although the higher temperatures in extrusion have a greater destructive effect on vitamins, the destruction of biological catalysts in the ingredients means that the stability of the vitamins in extruded diets after manufacture is actually higher than in pelleted food.

Dietary intake will be affected by the colour, smell and taste of the food. Most primate species prefer sweet foods. The hardness and density of the food will also affect intake, if it is too hard and uncomfortable to bite, then intake will decrease. The size of the food pieces needs to be small enough to be held easily as primates like to be able to manipulate their food. Some caretakers soak food in water to increase palatability but this is not to be recommended as it can lead to spoilage by moulds and bacteria, will reduce the vitamin content and can be detrimental to oral health.

Food may be offered *ad libitum* or given in a fixed amount. Primates eat to their energy requirements but can on occasion become obese if fed on palatable foods *ad libitum*, especially animals at the top of the social hierarchy who may monopolise favoured foods. Since the density of extruded diet may vary between manufacturers and between batches, it is unwise to feed by volume. Feeding should therefore be based on weight measurements for this type of diet.

ENERGY REQUIREMENTS

The gross energy (GE) of food is the total of the apparent digestible energy (DE) and the gross energy of the faeces. However the true DE is made up of the apparent DE minus the faecal metabolic energy losses, the gaseous energy losses, and heat of fermentation. The DE is not a constant but depends on food composition, food consumed per unit of time and the ability of the animal to process and digest it. The metabolisable energy (ME) is the total GE minus the GE lost in faeces, urine and gases. However, the diversity of primate species and the food items that they eat is so wide that the ME values for many food items in many primate species have not yet been determined.

An animal's energy requirement is the energy needed to support basal metabolic function, activity, maintenance of body temperature, product formation (tissue, growth etc.) plus the energy lost in faeces, urine, gases and heat. Smaller animals have a relatively higher basal metabolic rate, and energy expenditure is not dependent on the actual body weight (BW (kg)), but on the metabolic body weight, $(BW (kg)^{0.75})$, and the energy group to which the animal belongs (Wolfensohn & Lloyd 2003). Body composition also affects energy expenditure, a decrease in fat-free mass will lead to a decrease in basal metabolic rate. Therefore species, sex, age, growth, health, reproductive status will all affect energy requirements. It is therefore not possible to express food intake requirements accurately, simply in terms of food intake data expressed either as weight or energy, per kilogram body weight of the animal, since there is a very wide range of sizes of primates (35 g mouse lemur to 170 kg gorilla see Chapter 1) and a range of different body compositions.

The metabolisable energy contained in, for example, Old World monkey diet manufactured by SDS (Special Diet Services) is 2.85 kcal/kg, and the protein level is 19.5%. A healthy juvenile monkey weighing 2 kg needs 80–90 g diet daily (for energy), whereas an adult weighing 8 kg needs 110–190 g diet daily. This is intended as a guide only, and other factors such as reproductive status or health should be taken into account. Stressed, ill, pregnant or lactating animals may have greater needs. As practical guidance, each adult animal receives 100 kcal/kg/day, pregnant females 125 kcal/kg/day, lactating females 150 kcal/kg/day and growing juveniles 200 kcal/kg/day. This energy requirement is met by a combination of primate diet, a selection of fruit and vegetables and forage mix. The actual amounts will need to be adjusted according to the calorific value of the component parts. Commercial diets are formulated to be balanced, and animals receiving these quantities should be receiving sufficient protein, minerals and vitamins. However variety is an essential element of primate diet and when adding any supplements to the diet, such as fruit, care must be taken not to upset this balance. Amounts fed to animals will also need to be adjusted according to their activity and their weight gain/loss must be evaluated regularly.

CARBOHYDRATE, PROTEIN AND FAT

When formulating diets for non-human primates, the quantitative requirements for approximately 50 essential nutrients have to be considered. Diets are compounded from cereal mixes with protein, vitamin and mineral supplements, and many of the components will degrade over time, so care must be taken to ensure food is stored according the manufacturers instructions and not used after the expiry date.

Carbohydrate

Carbohydrates make up the majority of the components of plant material and provide 40% or more of the diet of most primate species. They are classified according to size: monosaccharides (simple sugars such as glucose), disaccharides (such as sucrose), oligosaccharides and polysaccharides. The polysaccharides are divided into starch, which can be digested by mammals, and non-starch, which is further divided into insoluble fibre and soluble fibre.

Table 4.1 Fibre concentrations in total dry matter of diets for primates placed into three groups aimed at the relative ability of three groups of primates to utilise plant cell wall (from NRC 2003a).

Fibre form and % dry matter	Examples of species
Group 1	
NDF 10	*Cebuella* spp.
ADF 5	*Callithrix* spp.
	Saguinus spp.
	Macaca spp.
Group 2	
NDF 20	*Pan troglodytes*
ADF 10	
Group 3	
NDF 30	*Propithecus* spp.
ADF 15	*Alouatta* spp.
	Colobus spp.
	Pygathrix nemaeus

NDF, neutral detergent fibre.
ADF, acid detergent fibre.

Inappropriate fibre intake can cause significant adverse effects in primates especially in species that have specialised fore- or hind-gut fermentation. The digestive capabilities of the primate species are related to their GI adaptations. Crude fibre (CF), which is found quantified on the feed packet, is the insoluble organic residue left after treatment with acid and alkali (to mimic digestion). However this process also causes solubilisation of the hemicellulose and lignin and is therefore a serious underestimate of the structural fibre content of the food. Hemicellulose cannot be digested by enzymes but needs fermentation and lignin is neither digested nor fermented. Although this error in the crude fibre determination is well recognised, the regulatory agencies still use it in feed analysis.

Nitrogen free extract (NFE) is also quantified on feed packets. This is the non-structural carbohydrate fraction which will therefore include varying amounts of the hemicellulose and lignin. It is better to define the physiologically functional component of total dietary fibres, which are the neutral detergent fibre (NDF), which includes the total insoluble fibre in the cell wall (primarily cellulose, hemicellulose and lignin), and the acid detergent fibre (ADF), which is primarily cellulose and lignin (the hemicellulose component therefore = NDF − ADF). It has been proposed that the fibre concentrations in total dry matter of diets for primates should be placed into three groups aimed at the relative ability of three groups of primates to utilise plant cell wall (see Table 4.1). These guidelines for diet formulations appear to be consistent with good health.

Protein

Most adult primates' protein requirement is less than 3 g/kg BW per day (4.6–7.5% ME calories or 6.4–8.0% dietary dry matter). The efficiency of protein use falls as the quality decreases and nutritional quality depends on amino acid composition, which must be a nutritionally balanced mixture. Protein from a single source should not be used, so combine grain and legume protein since each is limited in lysine and methionine respectively, or use animal and plant protein combinations to accomplish this. Most plant proteins are deficient in one or more of the amino acids methionine, lysine and tryptophan, whereas animal proteins have a better balance of amino acids. In diets in which much or all of the protein is derived from plant materials, it is important to use a mix of proteins to try to balance the amino acids. In complete primate diets, synthetic amino acids are often used to correct any remaining amino acid defiencies.

Fat

The essential fatty acids that cannot be made by the body in primates are the omega-3 and omega-6 fatty acids. In the rhesus, much of the brain development is achieved in the last third of pregnancy and the newborn brain is 70% of the adult weight. The omega-3 fatty acids are especially important in the diet of the pregnant female to ensure normal brain development in the offspring. There should be 1% ME (or about 0.5% by weight of dietary dry matter) as omega-3 fatty acids, represented by α–linolenic acid, to support normal development of the brain and nerve tissue. There should also be omega-6 fatty acid represented by 2% linoleic acid by weight in dry matter. Adequate dietary intake of the fatty acids is necessary for the absorption of the fat-soluble vitamins.

MINERALS AND VITAMINS

Minerals

The absolute requirements of different primate species are undefined but the major elements: calcium, phosphorus, magnesium, potassium, sodium, chlorine and sulphur; and the trace elements iron, copper, manganese, zinc, iodine, selenium, chromium and cobalt are required. There is possibly also a requirement for fluoride, molybdenum, silicon, boron, nickel, and tin.

Geophagia (soil eating) assists in obtaining the necessary trace elements, and clays have a role in neutralising phytotoxins in the diet. The bioavailability of the minerals should always be considered, since they may be bound – thus decreasing the amount actually available to the animal. For example, calcium bound to oxalate and phosphorus bound to phytate are largely unavailable to single-stomached animals. Some minerals may be toxic at relatively low levels, e.g. cadmium, lead, antimony, so care must be taken to avoid these.

Calcium and phosphorus are necessary for healthy bones and teeth and cellular function. Although there are skeletal reserves of both to offset short-term deficiencies, in the longer term, calcium deficiencies will lead to reduced growth, rickets, ostemalacia, and/or osteoporosis. Deficiencies in phosphorus can lead to poor growth, abnormal bones and teeth, and pica. It is necessary to provide at least 0.55% DM calcium. Many diets are provided to captive primates as nutritionally complete pellets plus fruit, vegetables and other treats. With this free choice there is an increased possibility of calcium deficiency since these supplements are either lacking calcium or the calcium is unavailable (e.g. in spinach it is bound to oxalate). If insects are fed to primates, the insects should be fed on

Table 4.2 Recommended concentrations of minerals.

Mineral	Concentration
Calcium	0.8%
Phosphorus	0.6%
Magnesium	0.08%
Potassium	0.4%
Sodium	0.2%
Chloride	0.2%
Iron	100 mg/kg
Copper	20 mg/kg
Manganese	20 mg/kg
Zinc	100 mg/kg
Iodine	0.35 mg/kg
Selenium	0.3 mg/kg

a calcium-rich diet for 2–3 days before use. The dietary Ca:P ratio should be in the range 1:1 to 2:1. Table 4.2 gives recommended concentrations of minerals.

Vitamins

Information on the vitamin requirements of primates is limited by available research data and species variations. However experiences of feeding commercial diets shows that they are probably not far off the required levels. It is worth noting that most manufacturers' data sheets express vitamins as those in the unprocessed meal (i.e. those added via a pre-mix and those vitamins naturally occurring in ingredients) and since most primate diets are extruded there can be significant subsequent losses. The levels of vitamins shown in Table 4.3 should therefore only be used as a guide.

WATER

Water distribution, intake and excretion are all affected by activity restriction, cold acclimatisation and water deprivation. In contrast to the amount of literature on consequences of calorific restriction, there is very little scientific evidence to specify the minimum fluid requirements of the different species. The amount of water drunk to satisfy physiological needs will depend on many factors such as the water and electrolyte content of the food eaten, the ambient temperature and humidity, and activity level of the animal. In the wild, most primates drink from running or standing water, and may use their hands or leaves, or lick moist rocks and plants. The mean total water intake in long-tailed macaques has been found to be 76 ± 35 ml/kg per day for males and 100 ± 51 ml/kg per day for females of which drinking water was 50 ± 33 ml/kg per day for males and 49 ± 48 ml/kg per day for females (Suzuki *et al.* 1989). Even moderate restriction of water source will reduce food consumption. Water quality can contribute to the mineral levels in the body, but this can also lead to toxic levels of some minerals if the levels in water are excessive.

Table 4.3 Recommended levels of vitamins.

Vitamin	Level	Comments
Vitamin A	12 000 IU/kgDM	Hypervitaminosis A can be as problematic as hypovitaminosis A, the correct balance is very important
Vitamin D	1000–3000 IU/kgDM	Required if the animal is not exposed to UVB radiation either from the sun or from artificial sources. It is preferable to provide this rather than supplement the vitamin as this will avoid potential problems due to overdosage
Vitamin E: (α-tocopherol)	50 mg/kgDM	
Vitamin K	2 μg/kg BW per day	
Thiamine	1.1 mg/kgDM	
Riboflavin	1.7 mg/kgDM	
Niacin	16–56 mg/kgDM	
Vitamin B6	4.4 mg/kgDM	
Biotin	110 μg/kgDM	
Folic acid	2.55–5.61 mg/kgDM	
Vitamin B12	11 μg/kgDM	
Vitamin C	55–110 mg/kgDM	Unless stable vitamin C has been used (e.g. Roche StayC, BASF LutavitC), this may be lost readily during storage or if the food is soaked to make it more palatable

Some neuroscience protocols in which primates are used, require the regulation of the animals' food or fluid intake. This regulation may simply involve strict scheduling of the access to water, or may involve restriction in which the total amount of water is strictly controlled, so that thirst becomes the motivator for performance of certain tasks. On such protocols the amount of fluid consumed and a hydration assessment should be recorded daily for each animal. Variables that can be used to assess hydration status include the body weight, food intake, skin turgor, urine output, moistness of faeces, general appearance and demeanour. Animals should generally be given free access to water for some period of time on days when there are no experimental sessions (NRC 2003b). There is currently much debate over the use of water restriction paradigms and guidelines have been issued by the UK Home Office (2002).

SUPPLEMENTS

Fruit, vegetables, insects and nutritionally complete treats are usually more palatable than pellets or extrusions (Figure 4.1). Care is therefore needed in their presentation to

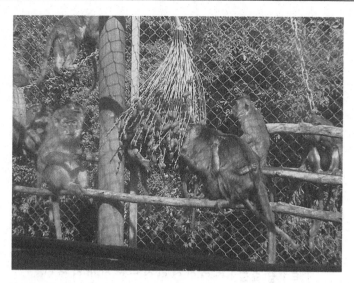

Figure 4.1 Feeding fruit.

ensure that the total diet does not end up nutritionally unbalanced. Supplements are generally given for environmental enrichment or as part of positive reinforcement training (see Chapter 7), rather then primarily for nutrition, but may have the undesired effect of distorting the nutrition provided. It is therefore important to use items that are nutritionally complete or are high in moisture and low in calories, such as fresh fruit and vegetables rather than offering energy dense but nutritionally incomplete foods such as nuts and raisins. Since fruit and vegetables are 80–90% moisture, if these make up less than 40% of the wet weight of the diet, they will be providing less than 10% of the total dietary dry matter and therefore will distort the nutrient balance only minimally.

Making use of texts that contain tables of composition of foods and feed ingredients with details of such data as dry matter, energy, protein level etc., is essential for formulating feeds and diets that will meet the requirements of primates. For example Table 4.4 shows examples of the nutrient content of some commonly used primate food supplements, both on an 'as fed' and dry matter basis (from Food Standards Agency 2002). The exact analysis of fruit will vary depending on the condition of the particular batch, the season and the source; but this table serves to demonstrate the relative values of common supplements and how these may affect the overall nutrition of the animals.

DIFFERENT LIFE STAGES

The requirements for different stages of development vary widely. Animals should be fed according to their individual needs, which depend on age, sex, physiological and reproductive status, health and environmental conditions. Estimates of energy requirements are usually related to the stage of development: maintenance, growth, pregnancy and lactation; often as some multiple of the maintenance requirement. For example, an adult may only need 25–50% of the energy needed by a juvenile which will have a smaller

Table 4.4 Examples of nutrient content of some commonly used primate food supplements.

	As fed basis						Dry matter basis				
	Moisture (g/100g)	Metabolisable energy (kcal/100g)	Crude protein (g/100g)	Crude fat (g/100g)	Vitamin C (mg/100g)	Dietary fibre (g/100g)	Metabolisable energy (kcal/100g)	Crude protein (g/100g)	Crude fat (g/100g)	Vitamin C (mg/100g)	Dietary fibre (g/100g)
Apple	84.5	47	0.4	0.1	6	1.8	303	2.6	0.6	38.7	11.6
Banana (flesh)	75.1	95	1.2	0.3	11	1.1	382	4.8	1.2	44.2	4.4
Broccoli	88.2	33	4.4	0.9	87	2.6	280	37.3	7.6	737.3	22.0
Brussels sprouts	84.3	42	3.5	1.4	115	4.1	268	22.3	8.9	732.5	26.1
Cabbage	90.1	26	1.7	0.4	49	2.4	263	17.2	4.0	494.9	24.2
Carrot	88.8	30	0.7	0.5	4	2.4	268	6.3	4.5	35.7	21.4
Celery	95.1	7	0.5	0.2	8	1.1	143	10.2	4.1	163.3	22.4
Grape	81.8	60	0.4	0.1	3	0.7	330	2.2	0.5	16.5	3.8
Grapefruit	89	30	0.8	0.1	36	1.3	273	7.3	0.9	327.3	11.8
Kiwifruit	84	49	1.1	0.5	59	1.9	306	6.9	3.1	368.8	11.9
Lettuce	95.1	14	0.8	0.5	5	0.9	286	16.3	10.2	102.0	18.4
Melon, honeydew	92.2	28	0.6	0.1	9	0.6	359	7.7	1.3	115.4	7.7
Orange	86.1	37	1.1	0.1	54	1.7	266	7.9	0.7	388.5	12.2

Parsnip	79.3	64	1.8	1.1	17	4.6	309	8.7	5.3	82.1	22.2
Peach	88.9	33	1	0.1	31	1.5	297	9.0	0.9	279.3	13.5
Pepper (sweet)	93.3	15	0.8	0.3	120	1.6	224	11.9	4.5	1791.0	23.9
Pineapple (flesh)	86.5	41	0.4	0.2	12	1.2	304	3.0	1.5	88.9	8.9
Raisins	13.2	272	2.1	0.4	1	2	313	2.4	0.5	1.2	2.3
Sesame seeds	4.6	598	18.2	58	0	7.9	627	19.1	60.8	0.0	8.3
Sunflower seeds	4.4	581	19.8	47.5	0	6	608	20.7	49.7	0.0	6.3
Sweet potato	73.7	87	1.2	0.3	23	2.4	331	4.6	1.1	87.5	9.1
Tomato	93.1	17	0.7	0.3	17	1	246	10.1	4.3	246.4	14.5
Watermelon	92.3	31	0.5	0.3	8	0.1	403	6.5	3.9	103.9	1.3
Harlan Teklad 2050*	10	270	20.9	5	80	18.46	300	23.2	5.6	88.9	20.5
Harlan Teklad 2055[†]	10	340	26.1	5.7	80	12.44	378	29.0	6.3	88.9	13.8

* Neutral detergent fibre: 9.5.
[†] Neutral detergent fibre: 7.6.
From Food Standards Agency (2002).

body weight but will be growing and be more active. As energy expenditure decreases with increase in age, so there is a decrease in energy requirement. Most growth occurs during a fairly linear phase of the so-called sigmoid growth curve. Each gram of protein deposited represents about 5.4 kcal net energy, and each gram of fat 9.1 kcal net energy. It has been shown that low birthweight infants have energy expenditure about 20% more than normal birthweight infants. Energy requirement also varies depending on the size of the species. In species with a shorter gestation, earlier weaning, larger litters and early sexual maturation, the energy goes to rapid development of physiological function rather than growth. Larger species put the energy into growth and have a longer period of dependence on the maternal investment in that growth. Infant New World primate species require 300–500 kcal gross energy/kg BW daily, whereas infant Old World primate species require 200–300 kcal gross energy/kg BW daily, and adult requirements are 30–50% lower than the requirement for growth.

At peak lactation, sucking mammalian young consume milk energy at 225 kcal/BW $(kg)^{0.83}$ per day. Although metabolic size across the species is taken as BW $(kg)^{0.75}$ (see page 46 in this chapter) this is a mathematical relationship which may not hold within one sub-group of mammals such as primates so other coefficients may be used for specific groups of animals. Over-consumption of calories by immature animals will lead to excess weight gain, affect age of sexual maturity and adult weight, and predispose to obesity. Energy requirements for pregnancy and lactation for non-human primates are undefined, but a 30% increase in energy requirement is estimated. Lactation is the most energetically demanding phase of reproduction. Primate milk is dilute (8.5–34.1% dry matter, energy range is 0.5–1.8 kcalGE/g) but there are differences in maternal milk composition which reflect the differences in care provide by different primate species. Strepsirhines that carry their young produce more dilute milk than those that leave their young unattended for long periods.

Growth can be measured in various ways such as body weight, crown–rump length, limb length, or head circumference. The linear measurements are not distorted by accumulations of body fat in the way that body weight may be. Growth rate will vary depending on genetic background, maternal nutrition in pregnancy and lactation, availability of supplementary weaning foods and rearing practices.

Milk composition varies throughout lactation (the concentration of fat and protein and the volume gradually decrease) and the time of sucking (the fat concentration is less at the beginning of a session than at the end). Human milk replacement formulas that provide ME at 0.67 kcal/ml, may be used successfully for primate rearing but may need to be supplemented with vitamin D. Transfer to solid food is easy at 2–4 months and older monkeys prefer to handle and chew food rather than drinking it. Age-related disorders are frequently linked to nutrition; dietary restriction (but without essential nutrient deficiencies) will increase survival and delay the onset of degenerative aging conditions. A persistently positive energy balance will lead to accumulations of adipose tissue with increasing body weight and obesity.

$$\text{Obesity index for rhesus} = \frac{\text{Weight (kg)}}{(\text{Crown–rump length (cm)})^2}$$

(Jen *et al.* 1985)

Social rank may be associated with obesity (Kemnitz 1984) since the dominant animal determines feeding time and the subordinates eat afterwards, depending on spatial distribution of food and the mix of food types. Chronic dietary restriction also protects against the development of insulin resistance in ageing rhesus monkeys, obesity is necessary for diabetes to develop in the rhesus although it is not the sole causal agent.

HAND REARING OF INFANTS

Sometimes it is necessary to hand rear infants, due to human interference or because of maternal neglect or death or because the mother has an inadequate supply of milk. In the latter case it may be possible to leave the infant with the mother for nurturing and care and simply to provide supplementary feeding until the animal is able to take food for itself. This is the preferred option since it will develop within its natal and peer group and the incidence of any consequential behavioural abnormalities will be reduced.

Once it has been established that an infant should be removed from its mother for hand rearing, it should be placed in a cage with some type of surrogate mother. This should be soft to touch, warm and if possible should move gently. The infant should be checked at least five times daily. Each day the infant's body weight is recorded and its physical state monitored. The parameters to be monitored include level of activity and general alertness, body tone, quality and quantity of faecal output, peripheral perfusion and weight gain. Hand feeding is not a precise activity and the timing of feeds and quantity of feed given may be varied according to the viability of the infant, but all information on the infant's food intake should be recorded.

The incidence of triplet and quadruplet births in marmosets has increased with improved standards of nutrition and health. The parents are rarely able to raise more than two offspring by themselves, so in such cases the offspring should be raised by rotational feeding (Figure 4.2), or only two should remain with the mother, the other being hand reared or euthanased promptly to avoid unnecessary suffering of rejection.

It may sometimes be necessary to foster or hand rear macaque young (Figure 4.3) but animals should not be maintained in isolation. In some cases they may subsequently be unsuitable for breeding but may facilitate human socialisation programmes.

Protocol for hand rearing

If a newborn infant is removed from the mother, it may be bathed in warm water and dried carefully but thoroughly. The first feed of glucose solution, usually 1–2 ml, should be offered as soon after bathing as possible. A weak infant may require a second glucose feed about an hour later. Approximately 1.5 hours after the first glucose solution feed and then every 1.5 hours, on the first day, infants are fed with milk formula, such as SMA, from a 5-ml syringe fitted with a rubber teat. Patience is necessary, the liquid must not be forced into the infant's mouth since attempting to feed quickly may result in fluid aspiration. Newborn animals should be checked and offered a feed in the evening and early morning to limit the hours between feeds. These feeds will continue until the infant begins to feed itself, which should be at around 10–14 days of age. The quantity of feed

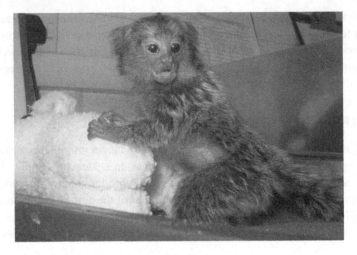

Figure 4.2   Bottle-fed marmoset on rotational feeding.

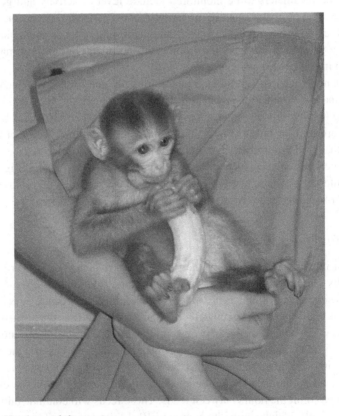

Figure 4.3   Hand-reared rhesus macaque.

will vary individually, but in the first 2 days, feeds of between 5 and 15 ml are normal. Those taking larger feeds will require fewer of them. The proportion of milk formula is gradually reduced, being replaced by semi-solid infant food as the animal learns to feed itself from a bowl. It is important to monitor health and weight gain during this changeover, by weighing the infant daily before feeding. A small reduction in weight from the birth-weight is normal but this is usually regained within 7–10 days. The infant may require cleaning or bathing each day, but ensure that it is dried thoroughly. Some infants learn to drink milk from a bowl very quickly, so milk formula can be provided in a plastic bowl during the first week. Night feeds can be eliminated once it is certain that the infant can feed itself from the bowl and that weight gain is being maintained. If the infant vomits or develops diarrhoea, the semi-solid infant food must be withdrawn from the feed and reintroduced after 2–3 days.

At 2–3 weeks most infant macaques are past the critical stage, and where possible should be paired with a peer. They will now make the most of an activity cage, which should be equipped with some play items. By 4–6 weeks, dry monkey pellets and diced fruit can be introduced as a novelty supplement to familiarise the animals with this type of food. Body weight can now be recorded every other day if there is no cause for concern. At about 2–3 months, Farex is added to the milk formula as an extra dietary supplement and to thicken it to start the adjustment to solid food. At 4 months, the infant macaque may be transferred to a large gang-style cage containing plenty of toys and climbing apparatus. Infants are then fed a complete dry primate diet with treat mix and fruit daily. Milk formulas may be given as a supplement only to the primate diet which is now given *ad libitum*. Body weight is now monitored weekly. Between 4 and 5 months, Farex can be removed from the diet and substituted with Complan. At 6 months, hand-reared infants can be considered, depending on individual weight, for mixing with naturally reared infants and little further intervention should be required apart from monitoring of behaviour. Care is needed to ensure the animal's psychological health is not damaged when it is reared artificially (see Chapter 6), but it is possible to hand rear infant macaques that go on to breed normally, despite much opinion to the contrary.

FURTHER READING

Chivers, D.J. & Hladik, C.M. (1980) Morphology of the gastrointestinal tract of primates: comparisons with other mammals in relation to diet. *Journal of Morphology*, **166**, 337–386.

Fleagle, J.G. (1999) *Primate Adaptation and Evolution*, 2nd edn. Academic Press, San Diego, California.

Food Standards Agency and Institute of Food Research (2002) *McCance and Widdowson's The Composition of Foods*, 6th edn. Royal Society of Chemistry, London.

The Home Office (2003) *Water and Food Restriction for Scientific Purposes*: Home Office Guidance Note. The Stationery Office, London.

Jen, K.L.C., Hansen, B.C. & Metzger, B.L. (1985) Adiposity, anthropometric measures and plasma insulin levels of rhesus monkeys. *International Journal of Obesity*, **17**, 597–604.

Kemnitz, J.W. (1984) Obesity in macaques: spontaneous and induced. *Advances in Veterinary Science and Comparative Medicine*, **28**, 81–114.

Lindburg, D.G. (1991) Ecological requirements of macaques. *Laboratory Animal Science*, **41**, 315–322.

Martin, R.D. (1990) *Primate Origins and Evolution.* Academic Press, New York.

NRC (1998) *The Psychological Well-Being of Nonhuman Primates.* National Research Council. National Academy Press, Washington D.C.

NRC (2003a) *Nutrient Requirements of Nonhuman Primates.* National Research Council. National Academy Press, Washington D.C.

NRC (2003b) *Guidelines for the Care and Use of Mammals in Neuroscience and Behavioural Research.* National Research Council. National Academy Press, Washington D.C.

Tardif, S., Jaquish, C., Layne, D., *et al.* (1998) Growth variation in common marmoset monkeys fed a purified diet: relation to care-giving and weaning behaviours. *Laboratory Animal Science,* **48**, 264–269.

Suzuki, M.T., Hamano, M., Cho, F. & Honjo, S. (1989) Food and water intake, urinary and faecal output, and urinalysis in the wild-originated cynomolgus monkey (*Macaca fascicularis*) under individually caged conditions. *Experimental Animal,* **38**, 71–74.

Wolfensohn, S.E. & Lloyd, M.H. (2003) *Handbook of Laboratory Animal Management and Welfare,* 3rd edn. Blackwell Science, Oxford.

Chapter 5
Physical well-being

The welfare of primates will be maximised by keeping the animals in good health. This applies not just to their physical health but also to their mental health (see Chapter 6). The health should be evaluated regularly and records kept and a programme to review and improve physical and mental health applied where necessary.

ASSESSMENT OF PHYSICAL HEALTH

The first step in carrying out a clinical examination to assess the monkey's physical health is simply to observe the animal in its home cage and evaluate its appearance, behaviour and general demeanour. To do this it is vital that the observer has some experience of the animal (both the species and the individual) in order to be able to judge whether the animal is exhibiting a normal behavioural repertoire. Just like humans some individual non-human primates will exhibit behavioural patterns that are specific for that individual, but do not necessarily reflect poor well-being. Note first the monkey's response to your presence. It may appear inquisitive or it may appear frightened or simply non-responsive. It may sit very still but be very aware of your presence and follow your every move with its eyes. A captive-bred macaque should interact well with its human carers and any changes in this behaviour should be investigated further.

Still without entering the enclosure, it should be possible to evaluate the animal's skin and fur condition. A loss of fur may indicate an underlying skin infection, which could be bacterial or parasitic or may be due to hair pulling. This over grooming, either by conspecifics or self-inflicted, frequently indicates an inadequacy of the environment resulting in boredom, or some other stress factor such as bullying by other animals. This may be from an animal in visual but not tactile contact. A rough estimate of body condition can be evaluated from a distance, as can its ability to walk, run, jump and to use all four limbs without signs of lameness or imbalance. The monkey will usually look at the observer and chatter, which is an opportunity to examine head and eye movements and to look at the condition of the front teeth and nostrils. Note any abnormal discharges or any unevenness or swellings. Remember the cheek pouches in the macaque may be full of food and therefore be uneven! Check again later to ensure the monkey has emptied them properly. If the monkey posterior presents, this will give an opportunity to inspect the external genitalia. Once a full and careful observation of the animal has been carried out, which needs time and patience and should not be hurried, look at the animal's enclosure.

Notice the condition of any substrate material and whether the monkey has had diarrhoea, or indeed has passed any faeces at all. When was the substrate last cleaned out? Is there evidence that the monkey has been playing with the substrate and the toys provided or do they seem to have been ignored showing that the animal is not, for some reason, exhibiting normal behaviour when you are not there. What food and drink are provided and has it been taking them? Is there evidence of urine production, is this excessive? If there are traces of blood around, look to see if the monkey is menstruating, the regular carer should have details of her cycle.

Monkeys will often appear to show little reaction to pain. A monkey in pain will have a generally miserable appearance, and may adopt a huddled position or crouch with head forwards and arms across the body. It will have a 'sad' expression with glassy eyes. It may moan or grunt, and tend to avoid companions. Grooming may stop, and food and drink are usually refused. Ill monkeys may attract extra attention from cage mates, varying from social grooming to attack. Acute abdominal pain may be shown by facial contortions, clenching of teeth, restlessness and shaking. Vocalisation is more likely to indicate anger than pain. Look at the monkey's companions. Are they all in a similar physical condition or is this one different in some way? A disease problem may be common to the whole group and all the animals may be affected in some way.

After completing the examination from a distance and noting the behavioural responses, only then should you catch the animal in order to look at it more closely. Catching it will markedly affect its behaviour, whether or not sedatives are used, which it why it is important to make a full evaluation first, before you disturb it any more than simply by your presence.

Quantitative assessment of well-being

Quantitative assessment of the animal's well-being can be usefully recorded with a clinical score sheet such as in Figure 5.1. This is a generalised all-purpose one. The animal should be reassessed at appropriate intervals in order to monitor its progress and check on the responses to any treatment given or changes in management that have been put in place. Often this type of all-purpose score sheet is too general to be sensitive enough to monitor these changes so it may be necessary to modify it to provide more specific information. An example of a sheet for monitoring a monkey with a neurological deficit is given in Figure 5.2 (Wolfensohn & Lloyd 2003). The general score sheet needs to be modified for each condition with which you are dealing, but once in place provides a very good way to monitor the animal. It is especially useful where more than one person is caring for the animal, in order to achieve consistency between carers. For monkeys used experimentally it also enables the setting of a humane endpoint by marking a score beyond which the animal will be euthanased to prevent suffering. Used in this way the clinical score sheet removes the variation of interpretation of clinical signs that is frequently found between animal care staff and research staff, and the criteria for intervention are clearly defined before the animal's condition deteriorates.

Clinical examination

In order to carry out a full examination of a primate it may be necessary to sedate it to reduce the risk of injury to the handler, to reduce the stress to the animal and also to enable the examination to be carried out thoroughly to yield the maximum possible information.

PARAMETER	ANIMAL ID:	SCORE	DATE/ TIME	DATE/ TIME
APPEARANCE	NORMAL	0		
	GENERAL LACK OF GROOMING	1		
	COAT STARING, OCULAR AND NASAL DISCHARGES	2		
	PILOERECTION, HUNCHED UP	3		
FOOD AND WATER INTAKE	NORMAL	0		
	UNCERTAIN: BODY WEIGHT↓<5%	1		
	↓ INTAKE: BODY WEIGHT ↓ 10–15%	2		
	NO FOOD OR WATER INTAKE	3		
CLINICAL SIGNS	NORMAL T, CARDIAC AND RESPIRATORY RATES	0		
	SLIGHT CHANGES	1		
	T ± 1°C, C/R RATES ↕ 30%	2		
	T ± 2°C, C/R RATES ↕ 50% OR VERY ↓	3		
NATURAL BEHAVIOUR	NORMAL	0		
	MINOR CHANGES	1		
	LESS MOBILE AND ALERT, ISOLATED	2		
	VOCALISATION, SELF-MUTILATION, RESTLESS OR STILL	3		
PROVOKED BEHAVIOUR	NORMAL	0		
	MINOR DEPRESSION OR EXAGGERATED RESPONSE	1		
	MODERATE CHANGE IN EXPECTED BEHAVIOUR	2		
	REACTS VIOLENTLY, OR VERY WEAK AND PRECOMATOSE	3		
SCORE	IF YOU HAVE SCORED A 3 MORE THAN ONCE, SCORE AN EXTRA POINT FOR EACH 3	2–5		
	TOTAL	0–20		

JUDGEMENT

0–4   Normal.
5–9   Monitor carefully, consider analgesics or other treatments.
10–14 Suffering, provide relief, observe regularly.
15–20 Severe distress, consider euthanasia.

Figure 5.1   General welfare assessment score sheet.

For smaller primates such as marmosets, manual restraint may be sufficient (see Figure 5.3), or may be used before then injecting a sedative by an appropriate route, usually intramuscularly. Larger primates, such as the rhesus macaque, may need to be sedated before handling or else they may cause physical injury to the handler. A restraint cage may be used for this, in which the back is pulled gently forward or the front pushed gently backwards.

ANIMAL NAME:							
Date							
Time							

Signs		Score						
Movements on entering room	None	3						
	Head only	2						
	Walking sluggishly	1						
	Normal	0						
Head posture on entering	Head pressing	2						
	Lowered	1						
	Normal	0						
Provoked behaviour	None	4						
	Blinking or frowning	3						
	Head lifting	2						
	Walks sluggishly	1						
	Normal	0						
Gait	Not moving	4						
	Hind leg dragging	3						
	Sluggish	1						
	Normal	0						
Ability to grasp	None	4						
	Sluggish	3						
	Normal	0						

Grooming	No	3					
	≤ once over 5 min	2					
	Decreased but > once	1					
	Normal	0					
Wounds	Discharge and swollen	3					
	Discharge or swollen	2					
	Sutures missing	1					
	Normal	0					
Eating	No	4					
	Takes small bits only	2					
	Takes larger bits	1					
	Normal	0					
Water consumption in the last 24 hours	None	4					
	None to 50% of normal	2					
	>50% of normal	1					
	Normal	0					
Total score							
Initials							

Comments:

Total score possible: 31

Action points: more than 6: provide treatment and relief

Assessor's Name/Contact details:

Figure 5.2   Neurological welfare assessment score sheet.

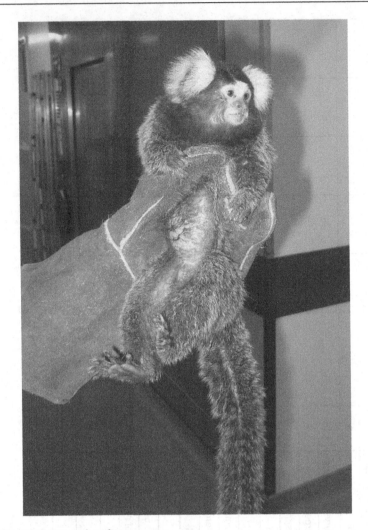

Figure 5.3   Manual restraint of a marmoset.

Matters of cage design to facilitate handling are discussed in Chapter 2. The animal may also be netted but this is a significant stress factor and most animals will not respond well to this method of capture. Much preferred is to spend time training the monkey to 'posterior present' for injection of sedative (see Figure 7.3) which can then be carried out with minimal stress to animal or handler.

Assessment of body condition

The animal's weight should be recorded and its body condition noted. This may be scored in a similar way to condition scoring of sheep (MAFF 1994). It is assessed by palpating the monkey over its thoracic and lumbar vertebrae (at the level of the last rib) and making a judgement as to the amount of fat and muscle covering the bony prominences of the vertebrae and giving a quantitative score as in Figures 5.4 and 5.5. Condition

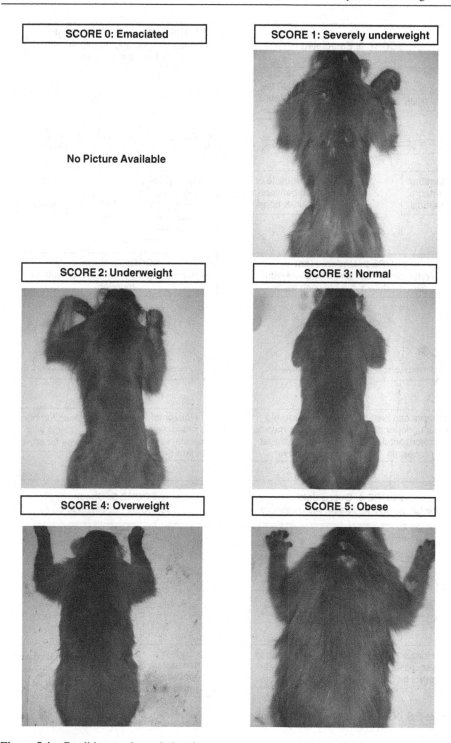

Figure 5.4   Condition scoring: whole primate.

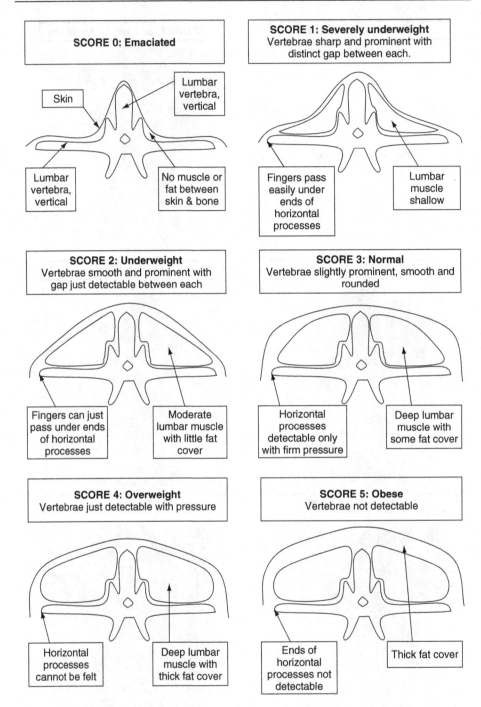

Figure 5.5 Condition scoring: vertebrae.

scoring at weaning and during the post-weaning period, combined with regular weight measurements, is important to ensure that the animal is receiving adequate nutrition and growing properly.

The clinical examination

Once the monkey's condition has been assessed, continue with the examination with it in dorsal recumbency. Hold the monkey's head and note that the eyes are straight with no discharge and that the pupils are even. Are the ears clean with no discharge and the pinna not swollen? Are the nostrils clean and even in size? Lift up the lips and note the colour of the gums, the condition of the incisor and canine teeth. Palpate around the jaw and throat noting any unusual swelling or any content in the cheek pouches. Gentle pressure on the angle of the jaw will enable you to open the mouth. Use an instrument such as a disposable tongue depressor or illuminated probe to then look inside the mouth, to examine the premolar and molar teeth, check the cheek pouches and the back of the throat. Never be tempted to put your fingers inside the mouth.

Run your hand down each arm and leg simultaneously checking for evenness in length and thickness of joints. Check the fingers and toes and trim the finger and toe nails if necessary in the same way as you would do your own. Observe the respiratory movements and palpate the abdomen gently. Examine the external genitalia and the anal and urethral orifices. Check the condition of the ischial pads in appropriate species and the tail, especially the tip.

Then take whatever samples are necessary for further investigations or as part of the colony health-screening programme.

QUARANTINE PROGRAMME

When acquiring new monkeys you will need some basic information to enable you to design your quarantine programme and then establish the health-screening programme. First consider the source of the animals. The choice of where you get the animals from will often be imposed simply by availability, but this will have profound effects on the design of your programme. How many animals do you want – and how many animals can your quarantine facility cope with at once? It might be better, and less risky, to bring in two smaller batches rather than one large one. This will be easier to manage and if there is a problem, it will reduce the risks.

Find out how were the animals kept in the source establishment, or were they of wild origin? Were they in peer groups or family groups? At what age were they weaned? If they were weaned young they will be more likely to be stressed and more likely to be carrying subclinical infections such as shigellosis, which may then become a clinical problem when they arrive. Were they housed indoors or outdoors? This will determine some infections to which they may have been exposed such as *Yersinia* from birds, or avian *Mycobacteria*, which may interfere with the interpretation of the tuberculin test.

What were the standards of care in the source establishment and the background health status of the source colony? Over what time period has this been established? Samples from individual animals may be meaningless in isolation from a full colony history.

If screening results are available, ask what test was carried out, where was the laboratory processing done, what was the quality control, were there any independent checks made?

Once you have decided where it is coming from, the monkey then has to be transported (see Chapter 9). How will this affect your health-screening programme? If it is only coming a short distance the effects of transportation will be much less of a problem than if it is coming half way round the world, stopping at airports in various countries where it may potentially encounter pathogens from other animals in airport holding areas. Find out how it is to be transported and what will be the prevailing environmental conditions. For example, if it travels miles in the back of a truck over bumpy ground in a large box there is likely to be muscle damage, but if it is in a small box with poor ventilation, there may be respiratory pathology after arrival. Will the monkey travel alone or with one of its peer group or with a stranger? These factors will influence the degree of stress placed upon it, may increase the likelihood of fight wounds, or of transmitting infections. All these parameters will influence your interpretation of signs you may see in the quarantine period.

Consider the husbandry conditions in the quarantine period. How will the incoming monkeys be isolated from existing stock? This could be in a different building, a separate area within the same building or, less ideal, simply a separate cage. Consider how to provide staff and manage their working practices so they do not risk spreading infection to existing stock (or *vice versa*). There should be adequate provision of protective clothing and changing areas, and methods to prevent spread of disease by rodents or insects. Who has access to these monkeys, and how soon after their arrival, will depend partly on their source. In a research establishment the scientist will often want to start work on the animal from the moment it arrives! However, it is vital to set aside enough time in programme planning for observation of these new animals, building up a picture of each one's normal behavioural repertoire, so that changes due to illness or experimental stress may be spotted rapidly. The key here is good quality staff and good technician training. It has been demonstrated that the behaviour of juvenile long-tailed macaques does not settle to pre-transport levels even 1 month after international transport and relocation to a new unit (Honess *et al.* 2004).

How long a primate should spend in quarantine also depends on the source. In the UK, under the Rabies (Importation of dogs, cats and other mammals) Order 1974, if it comes from overseas it will have to be held under rabies quarantine for 6 months. If there is any risk of filovirus, then an absolute minimum of 31 days quarantine should be applied. If there are doubts about simian herpesvirus (*Herpesvirus simiae*, B virus) and tuberculosis (TB) status then it will take 3 months to establish these. If the monkeys are from a source of which you can be 100% certain of the health status then you can move them sooner and quarantine then depends on the use to which they will be put.

HEALTH-SCREENING PROGRAMME

When considering clinical disease in primates it is obviously preferable to prevent disease states occurring rather than having to deal with them when they arise. In adddition, a number of infectious diseases of primates are potentially zoonotic, so a health-screening programme will not only improve the monkey's health and welfare and assist in the prevention of disease, but will also contribute to the occupational health programme of the institute in which they are kept (see Chapter 3).

Monkeys can carry a number of particularly pathogenic diseases, ranging from salmonellosis to tuberculosis, and the UK Advisory Committee on Dangerous Pathogens (ACDP) has made particular recommendations with respect to simian herpesvirus (*Herpesvirus simiae*, B virus), and simian retroviruses. For every facility holding primates a health-screening programme should be drawn up, which should take account of the source of the animals, the use to which they are put (e.g. breeding, experimental, zoo with public access), and the resources available for testing.

When designing a health-monitoring programme consider what samples to take, how many and how much to take and how the samples will be stored and then processed. Remember there are other sources of information available. All animals that die unexpectedly for whatever reason should be subjected to full post-mortem examination including routine monitoring of enteric organisms. A cause of death should be established on the basis of facts, not based on circumstantial and anecdotal evidence from care staff. In a research environment there may be plenty of available data from animals at the end of experiments. Take the opportunity to utilise this information and carry out a complete routine post-mortem examination (see page 71) on as many subjects as possible. Given the problems of false positives (and negatives) with tuberculin testing this may be a method of choice for screening for tuberculosis. The lungs may be examined for *Pneumonyssus simicola* (lung mites) (see Figure 5.6), and the bowel content cultured to keep a check on the normal bacterial flora. This is also sensible in order to check for changing antibiotic resistance, particularly if antibiotics are used routinely following experimental surgery. For example, if there is subclinical *Campylobacter* in the colony, it is useful to know the antibiotic sensitivity, so that if there is a clinical case treatment can be initiated promptly with an appropriate antibiotic.

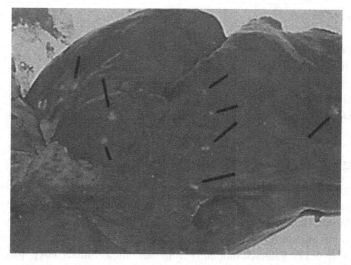

Figure 5.6   Lung damage due to *Pneumonyssus simicola*. Arrows indicate areas of scar tissue.

Random sampling for haematology, clinical biochemistry and faecal bacteriology and parasitology, will all yield useful background information about a colony. Ensuring a full investigation of any clinical disease may reveal background health problems that might be affecting the health of the colony, such as marginal nutritional deficiencies. There should also be in place an annual screening programme for selected diseases. As an absolute minimum, the Old World monkeys should have a screening history for B virus available and faecal bacteriology/parasitology should be carried out annually. Every such primate over 12 months of age should have the following carried out annually:

- serum sample to check BV serology (Old World monkeys)
- weight
- dentistry/oral examination
- fingers/toes/tail
- thoracic auscultation
- abdominal palpation
- other tests as necessary.

A regular health-screening programme will be maintained to cover some or all of the following:

- B virus
- simian immunodeficiency virus (SIV)
- simian T-lymphotropic virus (STLV-1)
- simian retrovirus (SRV-1, -2, -3)
- foamy virus
- hepatitis A
- Ebola
- Marburg
- tuberculosis
- faecal pathogens:
  - *Campylobacter*
  - *Salmonella*
  - *Shigella*
  - *Yersinia*
  - *Balantidium*
  - *Entamoeba*
  - *Trichuris*

Sampling strategy and reporting

The number of animals to be sampled (the sample size) should be appropriate for the pathogens under investigation, since the probability of detecting infection will depend on the infection rate (ILAR 1976; FELASA 1999). The minimum number for screening colonies or units should be 10, each unit being a self-contained microbiological entity. The samples should be gathered randomly from individual animals, not pooled. This will detect an infection incidence of 25–30% with a probability of 95%. In periodical routine investigations different animals should be used in succeeding tests. Serum samples for antibody testing should be taken from animals over 1 year in age, whereas faecal samples for bacteriology or parasitology will often yield more information when taken from juvenile animals.

The health monitoring report should contain information on:

- species, breed and unit to which the report applies
- date the colony was established
- list of organisms monitored
- date of latest investigation, diagnostic test used and identification of the testing laboratory
- results of latest investigation, number of positive/negative animals and number tested
- dates, test method, testing laboratory and results of the two preceding investigations
- any additional information of other investigations not included in the standard report such as investigations of sick animals.

Post-mortem procedure

Animals that have died should undergo a full post-mortem examination as soon as possible after death. If they are found out of normal working hours the carcase should be kept in a refrigerator at 4°C overnight, not frozen, so as not to damage tissues which may be required for histological examination, and then examined the following day. Carcases should be transported to the examining laboratory suitably bagged in clinical waste bags or in a clinical waste bin. A laboratory request form with details of the animal and any clinical history should accompany each carcase.

The weight of the animal is recorded; the animal should be weighed while in the bag and the weight of the bag deducted. The carcase is then placed into the Class I/III biological safety cabinet where it can be removed from the bags. All further procedures should take place in the safety cabinet.

Persons performing the post-mortem should wear suitable protective clothing; at least a laboratory coat, a non-absorbent apron, eye protection, nitrile gloves and waterproof sleeve covers. All surfaces should be kept as clean as possible during the post-mortem with any spillages of body fluids being cleaned up immediately. Disinfectant should be available at all times. Forceps should be used to handle tissues that are being cut.

The following post-mortem procedure is then performed.

1. The external appearance of the carcase should be examined with notes being made of its general condition and the presence of any lesions. All orifices should be examined for any abnormalities and discharges and a note made of any signs of vomiting or diarrhoea. Any samples from lesions or discharges should be collected at this stage.

2. Lay the animal on its back and swab the ventral surface with disinfectant (e.g. Virkon) to reduce contamination of internal tissues.

3. Make a midline incision from the chin to pubis and reflect the skin away from the incision line. The subcutaneous tissues and fat will need to be incised to reflect the skin.

4. The thorax should be opened first to reduce the risk of contamination from intestinal organisms. Hold the xiphisternum and cut laterally down just below the ribs, then cut

through the costochondral junctions on either side of the sternum. Reflect the sternum and ribs to expose the thoracic organs. Note any abnormalities such as the presence of pleural or pericardial fluid.

5. Remove the heart and lungs in order to make a more thorough examination noting any discoloration, adhesions or other abnormalities. Make incisions through the lung lobes and squeeze to see if there is any fluid present in the lungs. Open the heart by incising from the apex of the left ventricle into the left atrium and into the aorta, and from the apex of the right ventricle into the right atrium and into the pulmonary artery. Note any abnormalities of the heart valves and endocardium. Open the trachea lengthways and look for any inflammation or fluid. Tissues or swabs for microbiology should be collected aseptically into sterile containers and tissues for histology should be collected into 10% buffered formol saline.

6. Open the abdominal wall with a midline incision and reflect the wall sideways. Again note any obvious changes such as peritoneal fluid or liver abscesses.

7. Pull the intestine to one side and examine the urogenital tract and kidneys. Incise the kidneys longitudinally and inspect the internal structure. Examine the adrenal glands and reproductive organs.

8. Cut around the dorsal surface of the liver to remove it and cut through the lobes. Examine the cut surface for any abnormalities.

9. Remove the intestinal tract and examine its length, noting if the stomach is full or empty, whether there is any inflammation present, whether gas is present, and if the intestinal contents are fluid or solid. Examine the mesenteric lymph nodes.

10. If the clinical history indicates, examine the muscles, peripheral nerves, joints and bones.

11. If the clinical history indicates, remove the head, open the cranium and take out the brain for inspection.

12. All instruments used must be placed in disinfectant and thoroughly cleaned after use.

13. The carcase, tissues and other non-sharp waste must be placed into a clinical waste bin and sent for incineration. All syringes or sharps must be placed into a sharps bin and sent for incineration.

Equipment needed for post-mortem

- sterile pots and Petri dishes for the collection of tissues
- histology pots containing 10% buffered formol saline
- paper towels to mop up spillages
- disinfectant
- disinfectant discard jar
- scissors (various sizes)
- forceps: rat-toothed and dressing
- bone-cutting forceps

- scalpel handle and blades
- small bone saw
- trays

COMMON INFECTIOUS DISEASES

B virus

Cercopithicine herpesvirus type 1, also called herpesvirus simiae or simian herpes B virus, or most commonly BV, belongs to the simplex subfamily of the alphaherpesviruses. Virological and serological evidence demonstrates members of this subfamily are indigenous agents throughout primate species (Eberle & Hilliard 1995). BV infects the Asiatic macaque species, Simian Agent 8 (SA8) infects vervet monkey species, herpesvirus papio type 2 (HVP2) infects baboons, and herpesvirus tamarinus infects squirrel monkeys. Great apes have not been known to harbour B virus. These viruses are in the same sub-group as human herpes simplex virus (HSV).

Typically, in the natural host, simplex-like viruses cause a mild or inapparent disease, although in other species disease may be severe. BV has caused at least 40 cases of disease in humans, most of which (70%) were fatal (Holmes *et al.* 1995), almost all of them from occupational exposure to laboratory primates. Infection is lifelong with viruses adopting latent state in sensory ganglia and periodic reactivation from latency occurs as a result of physiological or immunological stress. Clinical signs in monkeys parallel herpes simplex virus in man; in rhesus, primary infection in young animals is usually unnoticed with minor buccal ulceration observed on few occasions whereas in long-tailed macaques, primary infection has not been reported as obviously symptomatic. The natural history of BV in monkeys shows similarities with herpes simplex in man but there are some distinct differences. The virus replicates at the entry point then migrates to the nerve ending and then establishes latent infection in the ganglia of the sensory nerves of the trigeminal nerve serving the oral cavity and the sacral ganglia serving the genital tract. Reactivation results in virus shedding without any further clinical signs.

Precise stimuli for BV reactivation and transmission remain to be defined; however, as with HSV, immunosuppression is an effective stimulus (Chellman *et al.* 1992). Weir *et al.* (1993) found that shedding of BV from seropositive macaques is uncommon when they are subjected to common laboratory procedures or environments, and that transmission is rare in singly housed animals. A number of studies have described a low frequency of BV isolation from seropositive macaques. However, it remains unclear if this low isolation rate reflects infrequent shedding or technical difficulties in primary culture of BV. Studies of experimental infections have demonstrated that virus shedding can be detected by polymerase chain reaction (PCR) when virus isolation by traditional methods has been unsuccessful (Slomka *et al.* 1993). This data and colony seroepidemiological studies would support very frequent shedding of BV from infected macaques. The incidence of BV infection, as estimated by isolations from genital tissues and their associated ganglia, appears highest around puberty, leading some researchers to conclude that the transmission is venereal (Zwartouw *et al.* 1984). However this conclusion may be confounded by the possible risk factors that routinely occur in conjunction with breeding activity such as grooming and aggression. In one 16-month study of 157 animals (Weigler *et al.* 1993), the data indicated that cage mate aggression was the primary risk factor for BV infection. Those monkeys that were bitten and scratched were nearly five times more likely to become infected during the same time period than monkeys that were not attacked. Male and female monkeys were at equal risk of infection in group-housed facilities and social dominance rank did not predict risk of BV infection. A recent PCR-based study of a rhesus macaque colony, which examined the ganglionic sites of BV latency, concluded that while sexual contact was significant it was not the predominant mode of transmission between monkeys (Weigler *et al.* 1995).

Zoonotic information

BV is spread to man by bites, abrasions contaminated with saliva and also aerosols entering by conjunctiva, nose and pharynx. There has been one reported case of human-to-human transmission (Weigler 1992). The clinical signs in man are that it is a highly fatal disease (mortality more than 70%) due to encephalomyelitis. The incubation period is not well documented but is approximately 1–5 weeks from exposure. Treatment with acyclovir has been used with some success. Human infection with BV is also multi-factorial with the sporadic nature of human case reports complicating efforts to quantitatively assess different risk elements of the causal pathway. Monkey-to-human transmission of the agent requires the presence of infectious titres of virus in monkey tissues or fluids presented in such a manner that allows replication in the human host, a particular set of circumstances which is unpredictable for any individual encounter. However the number of such cases should warn us to take precautionary measures at all times and to heed guidelines concerning testing and follow-up to exposures. Screening serum from staff for herpes simplex type 1 antibody is irrelevant since this does not protect against BV infection.

Diagnosis

In man diagnosis is usually achieved post-mortem by virus isolation from the brain, or if there is time, then antibody levels can be measured. However there is usually insufficient time for the titre to rise before death occurs. In the monkey, diagnosis is by clinical signs in the primary infection with or without virus isolation, and then serology. The appearance of ulcers (if they occur at all) can be primary or a secondary infection following reactivation, although the latter is infrequently seen.

In view of the high pathogenicity of BV in non-macaque primates, the UK Advisory Committee on Dangerous Pathogens has recently reclassified BV into hazard group 4 (ACDP 1998). In the event of an animal being diagnosed as seropositive it strongly advises that such an animal is destroyed and incinerated. If this is not done then the animal should be handled at full animal containment level 4, which would also involve consideration of the animal's welfare requirements. The guidelines also advise that negative results from sexually immature macaques should be regarded with caution as latent infection may be present and may be reactivated by stress or immunosuppression (Wolfensohn & Gopal 2001). It recommends that a representative sample of Old World monkeys held long term in any facility should be tested annually and in the event of a seropositive animal being found, the rest of the colony should be tested and the appropriate action taken.

Problems with BV serology

The group 1 herpesviruses are all closely related serologically (HSV, BV, SA8, baboon HV) and therefore cross reactions occur. Correspondingly, there are extensive cross-reactive antibody responses between the different viruses of the subfamily of alphaherpesviruses. Serum neutralisation antibodies persist for 6 months with progressive decay, so it is possible to have antibody-negative animals and yet detect traces of BV DNA. Production of antibody in the primary infection does not always occur and in very stressed animals there may be no antibody response owing to immunosuppression. In experimental infections ulcers appear 3–8 days after inoculation and seroconversion occurs at day 8–17. The antibody level is variable and depends on the diagnostic test used. If toxicology experiments are being carried out using immunosuppressive drugs, these can reactivate latent BV infection.

Diagnostic methods

1. *Virology*: The ulcer should be biopsied at post-mortem for histology and viral identification and culture. Scrapings from the mucosa may demonstrate virus before the ulcers are seen, therefore this is more accurate much sooner than serology, which does not become positive until later. The sample is cultured in monkey kidney cells and cytopathic effect is seen in 1–3 days. In order to avoid the culture methods that are time consuming and involve safety considerations, polymerase chain reaction (PCR) may be used in preference to detect the nucleated sequence of virus in studied cells. This is best used after a biting incident to indicate whether infection is present, but specific probes are not very efficient at binding. It is therefore usual to use a less specific probe and then cross check it against HSV to check that it is not that infection. This therefore allows detection of seronegative animals that are excreting virus. PCR can also be used to find latent virus in ganglia and so is useful for epidemiological studies.

2. *Serology*: The interpretation of a certain level of antibody detected is ambiguous because it can increase *without* a corresponding excretion of virus, or the antibody level can be high in the primary infection but not reach the same level during reactivation, or virus can be propagated *before* seroconversion, or some animals show no detectable humoral immune response.

It therefore becomes necessary to examine not just the serology, but also to look for virus from the monkey to be certain about its status. Even if an animal is seronegative, there will be uncertainty if it comes from an endemic zone because it could have been infected recently and not yet developed antibody; or it could have had antibody but the level is now decreased; or it may not have the virus and be genuinely negative. Therefore serology alone is only of use in a known epidemiological context rather than for the prevention of introduction of virus from monkeys where status is unknown.

Serological methods

1. *Competitive radioimmunoassay (RIA) test*: Primary screening for BV antibodies may be done by competitive radioimmunoassay (compria). Briefly, sera are tested for the ability to compete the binding of a BV-positive reference serum on a BV-infected cell antigen. Results are expressed as percentage inhibition of binding of mouse serum compared with an antibody-negative monkey pool. A rate of 0–30% binding is interpreted as a negative, 30–60% binding is equivocal and 60–100% is positive (Norcott & Brown 1993).

2. *Serum neutralisation test*: Compria positivity is confirmed by serum neutralisation (SN) of BV infectivity. Serum neutralisation titres are evaluated by reacting serial dilutions of sera with a constant viral inoculum (100 TCID50 where TCID50 = the 50% tissue culture infectious dose). A serum is regarded as being seronegative if it fails to neutralise approximately 100 TCID50 of the appropriate virus at a dilution of 1 in 2. For BV, seronegativity should be demonstrated against both BV and HSV.

3. *ELISA and Western blotting (WB)*: ELISA is generally used first as it is more sensitive and then Western blotting is used for better specificity. However if the specificity is increased too much this may lead to false negatives, if there are different BV strains, as some may not then be detected at all.

Recommendation

Screening for BV is therefore advised, using SN/RIA serology combined with ELISA and WB to avoid non-specific reactions. For investigations of individuals involved in specific incidents virological screens should be carried out on swabs from the animal's genitalia and mouth to reveal if the monkey transmitted virus at a bite. Animals used in experiments should wherever possible be from BV-free colonies or seronegative to BV, particularly where animals are handled under conditions of close contact, in long-term studies or for neurological surgery, or for work where a latent infection may be reactivated. Examples of such procedures are those involving psychological stress or immunosuppression, the establishment of tissue culture or cell lines, surgery of the brain or oropharyngeal region, the genital region or the neural ganglia related to these areas. Overall, the data suggest that although immunosuppression may lead to BV reactivation and shedding, 'normal' stimuli within the colony will result in frequent reactivation and transmission of infection. A serological screening programme will therefore rapidly detect the presence of BV-infected animals within a colony. The criterion for seronegative status is that each animal has a negative test for BV antibody on two occasions separated by at least 2 months, during which it is kept isolated from other monkeys who may be carrying the virus. Such a seronegative animal has a very low probability of carrying latent BV infection, although serological tests do not provide absolute freedom from infection.

A comprehensive programme of testing in the source colony over many years will enable one to interpret the results in individual animals from that source colony with more confidence. Unless full background information is provided, testing of single specimens may not be diagnostic and interpretation of the result is not possible (Kalter *et al.* 1997).

The animals should come from regularly monitored BV-negative stocks, from breeding colonies that are free of BV or their status should be confirmed by serologically testing each animal. All animals used to start a breeding colony should be screened. All Old World primates should be tested annually, the duration of maternal antibody is not well established, so interpretation of results from animals under one year may not be clearcut. All incidents should be taken seriously and guidelines should be in place to deal with potential transmissions of infection.

Simian retroviruses

The retroviruses are classified as oncoviruses, foamy viruses and lentiviruses and all of them have some significance in non-human primates, see Figure 5.7.

Oncoviruses

The type C oncoviruses include the human T-cell leukaemia viruses HTLV-1 and -2 and their simian counterpart STLV-1. Type D oncoviruses include feline leukaemia virus and macaque type D retrovirus, which can produce subclinical infection and slowly developing tumours as well as immunosuppression. These simian retroviruses (SRV) have been associated with immunodeficiency and wasting syndromes called simian AIDS with opportunistic infections and gingivitis. PCR is more sensitive for picking up SRV-D infections compared with virus isolation or, more importantly, serological screening (Lerche 1997). Antibodies to simian retrovirus D have been found to be present in many

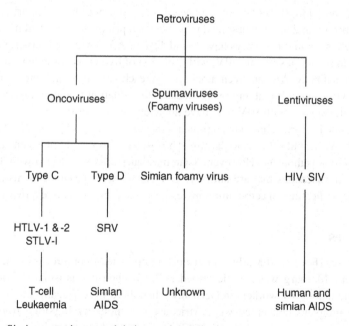

Figure 5.7   Simian retroviruses and their associated diseases.

African and Asian primates. Colony-born animals have a lower prevalence than wild-caught animals, but overall 3–4% of rhesus macaques may be seropositive, and up to 36% of long-tailed macaques.

Spumavirus (foamy virus)

Natural spumavirus infection in non-human primates does not apparently cause disease, although the prevalence of seroreactivity is high. Antibody is detected by PCR and the level remains stable. Simian foamy virus infection was found in 1.3% of animal care workers exposed to non-human primates (3 of 231). Seropositivity has not been found in people who are not exposed to non-human primates (sample of approximately 8000 people). However the risk of the development of disease in persons infected with these viruses remains undefined, although current thinking is that they do not pose a problem for human health, since there are now many years of data on seropositive humans and their sexual partners with no evidence of transmission or disease (Centers for Disease Control 1997).

Lentiviruses

The lentiviruses are not oncogenic but produce long-term persistent infections which lead to chronic debilitating diseases. This group includes HIV and simian immunodeficiency viruses (SIVs) well as the ungulate lentiviruses such as maedi-visna of sheep. Note that simian AIDS can be caused by both type D retroviruses and lentiviruses. It is important to be sure which is being described when reading accounts of a particular syndrome or disease pattern. There have been reports of seroconversion in laboratory workers who have been exposed to SIV either through needle-stick injury or by not wearing gloves.

SIV has been found to be widespread in non-human primates in the wild in areas where human AIDS is common. Surveys have found 42% of African green (vervet) monkeys in these areas to be seropositive for SIV, with isolation of live virus possible from almost all animals with antibody. African green monkeys can reach very high viral titres, with actively replicating virus, but without any overt illness. This situation is apparently analogous to that of people infected with HIV who have no symptoms of AIDS.

SIV infection in African non-human primates therefore produces high levels of circulating antibody and virus, but little or no disease. The virus passes readily between animals, but is apparently non-pathogenic. However, Asian macaques actively infected with SIV rapidly become ill. In macaques that are antibody positive but asymptomatic, virus isolation is not possible, indicating an active immune response suppressing viral expression.

Filoviruses

The filoviruses (Ebola and Marburg) have been implicated in outbreaks of fatal haemorrhagic fevers. Marburg was first described in 1967 when it was isolated from monkey handlers and laboratory workers in Germany when there were 7 deaths out of 31 human cases. The monkeys concerned were African green monkeys imported from Uganda. Ebola was first described in Africa in 1976 and there is high mortality associated with the human disease. This disease has received extensive press coverage in recent years as outbreaks have hit regions of Africa. Several strains of Ebola are now recognised, Ebola Zaire and Ebola Sudan are both associated with high mortality in humans. Ebola Tai Forest was found in the Ivory Coast in 1994 when a Swiss zoologist performed an autopsy on a chimpanzee and was infected with a non-fatal Ebola Tai Forest strain. Since then however, there have been more cases and some fatalities with this strain. In 1989 in Reston, Virginia a group of long-tailed macaques imported from the Philippines became ill with haemorrhagic disease, indicating a potential Asian focus for these viruses. Twelve primates in two of the 22 holding rooms became ill, the remainder were all put down. *The Hot Zone* (1994) by Richard Preston describes the 1989 outbreak in graphic detail and a film *Outbreak* was very loosely based on the story. None of the 149 people who came into contact with the animals or their tissues became ill, but four technicians showed seroconversion against the same strain of the virus. Further cases occurred and the common factor was that all the monkeys came from the same breeding farm in the Philippines.

The host and the natural transmission cycle for these viruses still remain unclear. Serological evidence shows that around 10% of the long-tailed, rhesus, and African green (vervet) monkeys coming into the USA from either Africa or Asia show serological evidence of filovirus infection. Around 5% of monkey handlers in USA and South-east Asia showed the presence of antibodies and also 2.7% of adults in the US who had no history of contact with primates also had a positive result for presence of antibodies. There is some difficulty in the interpretation of low antibody titres in the monkey. It is important to realise that Ebola causes an acute self-limiting infection and virus has not been isolated more than 20 days after onset of infection and never in the presence of significant antibody titres. Thus an antibody-positive animal is not infectious, the presence of the antibody simply indicates past exposure to the virus or related antigens. Therefore a quarantine period of 31 days is recommended. Signs of illness that warrant immediate investigation and containment are diarrhoea with melaena or frank blood, bleeding from external orifices, petechial haemorrhages or sudden death.

The ecology of the filoviruses remains obscure. Are they primate viruses that only cause disease in a small proportion of cases, or when they cross the species barrier; or do they have an as yet unidentified primary host with a wide geographical range? (For a full review see Schou & Hansen 2000.)

Tuberculosis

This is due to either *Mycobacterium tuberculosis* or *M. bovis*. It does not occur naturally in primates and outbreaks are generally caught initially from humans and then spread within non-human primate populations. The incidence of human tuberculosis is increasing, both in the UK and the USA, and visitors and keepers can be a source of infection for the animals. It is a significant zoonosis and care must be taken in handling any animal that is suspected of carrying the disease. Usually the source of infection can be traced to a recently imported animal or an infected human that has had contact with the colony. Infection occurs via the inhalation route, occasionally by digestion. The disease progresses slowly, taking up to one year to cause death in a rhesus. Clinical signs may be absent until the disease has become advanced, the most common sign is a cough. Apes are more susceptible to the disease than macaques, which are more susceptible than African monkeys, which in turn are more susceptible than New World monkeys. Tuberculosis causes a chronic progressive fatal disease in monkeys, and can pass from monkey to man and *vice versa*. The disease in monkeys can remain subclinical for 6 months or more, and indeed may be latent until the animal is terminally ill. To prevent the disease from entering the colony, all new animals should come with a health profile that indicates they have had at least three negative tuberculin tests before arrival, or they should be quarantined and screened on arrival. Any animal that has contacted a known human case should be effectively quarantined for at least 6 months until it is proved not to have contracted the disease.

The key to controlling tuberculosis is preventing it from getting into the colony in the first place, for which an effective quarantine programme and control of visitors who may be carrying TB is essential. Personnel intending to work with monkeys should be given the BCG vaccination or have their immunity checked using a Mantoux or Heaf test. To control or prevent an outbreak it is important to detect infected animals as early as possible. A screening test may be carried out using an intradermal (i.d.) skin test, and a useful site for this is the skin of the eyelid. Since an infected animal will be transmitting infected droplets to other animals within the first 3 weeks of becoming infected, it becomes very difficult to control an outbreak once it has started. Vaccination with BCG is generally inappropriate for non-human primates as protection only lasts for a few months and any usefulness of the tuberculin test for diagnosis will then be lost. Therapy may only suppress the disease without eradicating it, so the animal may then start to shed organisms again and continue to be a source of infection.

A 90-day quarantine with *at least three* tuberculin tests is the method of choice where possible, with all new arrivals having a thoracic radiograph taken on arrival and just before release, in order to detect advanced cases in which the animal may be anergic and give a false negative on the tuberculin test. This scheme may be modified according to individual circumstances, for example depending on the source of the animals and the perceived risk of their carrying infection.

The procedure for the i.d. tuberculin test is to tranquilise the animal and inject intra-dermally into the upper lid of the left eye, mid way between the medial and lateral canthi, 0.1 ml of a solution containing 1250 IU mammalian purified protein derivative (PPD) tuberculin in sterile water, which is prepared from *Mycobacterium tuberculosis*. A new 27 or 25G needle is used for each injection which is made as near as possible to the lid margin in order to raise a skin bleb (see Figure 5.8). The animals are then checked at 8, 24, 48 and 72 hours following injection and are scored according to Figure 5.9.

The test relies on the development of delayed hypersensitivity against a peptide contained in the mycobacterial cell. This delayed hypersensitivity develops in non-human primates 3–4 weeks after infection. This protein fraction in the tubercle bacillus and in the tuberculin is recognised by sensitised T lymphocytes causing release of lymphokines, local oedema and local cellular infiltration. An accurate response will therefore depend on a certain number of tubercle bacilli, sufficient circulating T cells and an adequate amount of specific antigen in the tuberculin.

Instead of mammalian PPD tuberculin, it is possible to use Koch's old tuberculin (old TB), which is the unfractionated heated concentrates of culture filtrates of mycobacteria

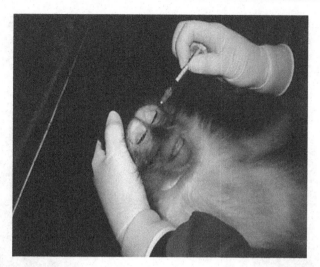

Figure 5.8   Intradermal injection of tuberculin.

0 = No reaction	⟶	Negative
1 = Bruise	⟶	Negative
2 = Erythema of palpebrum, no swelling	⟶	Negative
3 = Erythema of palpebrum and slight swelling	⟶	Positive
4 = Swelling of palpebrum, drooped eyelid and erythema	⟶	Positive
5 = Swelling and/or necrosis, eyelid closed	⟶	Positive

Figure 5.9   Classification of tuberculin test reaction. See Figures 5.10a and 5.10b.

grown in liquid media; whereas the purified protein derivatives (PPD) are precipitated fractions of culture filtrates. In non-human primates, old TB has greater reactivity than PPD so will be more sensitive, but leads to an increased incidence of false positive reactions. Old TB is almost impossible to obtain in the UK, although it may be possible to get it in other countries.

False positives and negatives occur quite frequently and complicate the interpretation of results, particularly if the TB test has been applied to specific valuable individual animals rather than to a whole batch with a similar history. False positives may be due to:

- use of buffered diluents instead of sterile water for diluting the tuberculin
- impurities in the tuberculin (especially Koch's old TB)
- trauma due to poor injection technique
- previous BCG vaccination
- cross reactions with atypical or saprophytic mycobacteria which share some antigens.

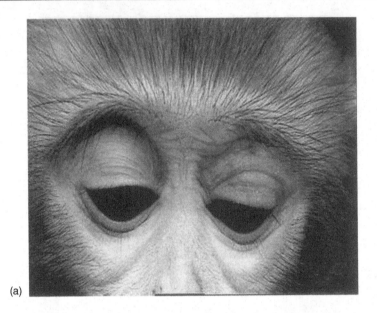

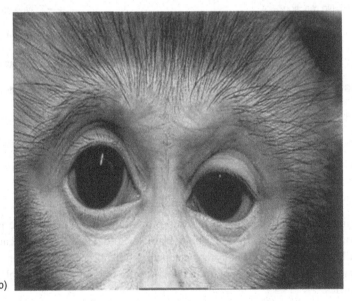

Figure 5.10   (a) Rhesus monkey tuberculin test score 3 and (b) Rhesus monkey tuberculin test score 4.

If a cross reaction is suspected, the test can be repeated and avian tuberculin included.
 False negatives may be due to:

● anergy due to overwhelming pulmonary tuberculosis
● testing early in infection before development of hypersensitivity
● systemic fungal disease

- concurrent measles infection or vaccination
- technical errors
- localised densensitisation if the test is repeated in the same site.

If anergy suspected, the test should be read at 2 and 8 hours as there may be a 'flash' reaction which is gone by 24 hours. The test can be supported by the use of radiography as the hilar lymph nodes are frequently an early site of the disease, but the heart shadow makes diagnosis difficult unless there is widely disseminated pulmonary disease. Culture of tracheobronchial washings is possible but not reliable. Polymerase chain reaction (PCR) can be used to detect bacterial DNA from samples, which has the advantage of being much quicker than the conventional culture methods of diagnosis. The modified PRIMAGAM^{TM} Rtest will detect γ interferon produced in response to stimulation of lymphocytes and can be useful to differentiate false positives due to cross reactions to antigens from different mycobacteria. Serological testing with an immunofluorescent antibody (IFA) test may be used to demonstrate humoral antibody response but the humoral immunity is far less sensitive than the cell-mediated immunity, limiting its usefulness. Recent work has shown the detection of early secretory antigenic target-6 antibody (ESAT-6) by ELISA may be a useful diagnostic tool (Brusasca *et al.* 2003; Kanaujia *et al.* 2003) for development of immunodiagnostics for tuberculosis. This will be more reliable than the interpretation of intrapalpebral testing for early diagnosis, which is so important in the management of primate colonies.

In summary the important points about tuberculosis in primates are:

- Skin tests are not 100% reliable.
- Infectivity precedes radiographic or clinical signs or positive tuberculin test.
- Radiographic signs precede clinical signs.
- Coughing is the most common clinical sign.
- No single test is reliable – use combinations.
- Take sequential chest X-rays of coughing monkeys.
- Routine post-mortem examinations will add to the available screening data.

Rabies

Animals imported into the UK will need to be subjected to rabies quarantine, and any personnel intending to work with such animals will need to be vaccinated against rabies. The occurrence of rabies in captive-bred monkeys is extremely rare but potential exposures do occur and given the serious zoonotic potential of the virus it should be taken seriously. Both the furious and the paralytic form have been seen in a range of species. The former develops in 15–35 days, the latter may take more than 100 days. The signs are variable and may include self-mutilation, irritability and paralysis of pharyngeal muscles.

Measles

Old World monkeys are susceptible to measles (Kobune *et al.* 1996), and may be vaccinated against this at weaning. It is possible to use canine distemper virus vaccine, which shares the same antigens but this is now difficult to obtain without it being in combination with a range of other canine vaccines. The use of these in the primate has to be evaluated on a case-by-case basis as there is a risk of cross reactions and if the primate is to be used experimentally vaccination may interfere with the experimental results, particularly in the field of immunology. Human measles vaccines also come in combination with other antigens which it may be inappropriate to use in the non-human primate in some circumstances. The principle source of infection to the primate will be from contact with humans so it is advisable to limit the contact with humans whose antibody status to measles is unknown. Since the human vaccine to measles is widely available it is anticipated that the incidence of the disease will fall, particularly if uptake in children can be increased. This has fallen in recent years owing to the vaccine's combination with the rubella antigen, the supposed side effects of which have received an amount of adverse publicity.

Hepatitis viruses

Hepatitis A

Both humans and non-human primates are a reservoir for this enterovirus, although infection may be inapparent. Transmission is by the faecal–oral route and there have been several cases of primate-to-human infection reported. Vaccination for humans is readily available.

Hepatitis B

The apes are susceptible to this infection but usually asymptomatic. In humans the infection can have serious consequences, vaccination is available. Macaques do not carry hepatitis B.

Hepatitis C

Spontaneous infections in primates have not been reported although they can be infected experimentally.

SV-40 Papovavirus

This infection is widespread in rhesus macaques and there are no clinical signs, but there are possible implications in tumours in humans who have received polio vaccines derived from primates that were carrying the virus. It may therefore be necessary to include this virus in a health-screening programme for primates used in immunological research.

Monkeypox

There is an increasing incidence of human infection with this virus in Africa. A suggested reason for this is that, since smallpox has been eradicated, the human population has no smallpox immunity, which also provided some protection against monkeypox. The human population is therefore now more susceptible to this disease. This may have an effect on the pattern of disease seen in monkeys in due course.

Enteric disease

Enteric disease may be caused by a number of factors including pathogenic organisms. Monkeys will pass loose stools if they are frightened, or if there are changes in their environment or diet. Stresses such as these can also cause subclinical infections to become clinical, so any case of diarrhoea should be investigated to eliminate infectious causes. Zoonoses such as *Shigella*, *Salmonella*, *Campylobacter* and *Yersinia* are common bacterial pathogens, and protozoa such as *Entamoeba*, *Balantidium* or helminth parasites may also pose a risk. Some of these organisms can cause explosive outbreaks of disease and death if not controlled immediately. Regular screening and treatment will reduce the level of infection, and must be combined with strict hygiene and good husbandry to prevent transmission between animals and to personnel. Husbandry and environmental factors may also contribute to the development of enteric disease, as will the presence of parasites or viruses such as rotavirus, retroviruses and haemorrhagic viruses. Therefore, prompt and accurate diagnosis of the aetiology of the enteritis is important so that a specific therapy can be instituted.

Shigella infection

Shigellosis has long been recognised as a problem in non-human primates that have been newly imported and in those that have been stressed in some way. The disease spectrum can vary from a fatal peracute infection to the establishment of symptomless carriers that may shed organisms and act as a reservoir of infection. In these animals stressful events may convert a sub-clinical infection to clinical disease (Weil *et al.* 1971). As well as causing severe illness or death in monkeys, the infection is of concern because it is an important zoonosis (Kennedy *et al.* 1992), although proper procedures should be sufficient to prevent spread of shigellosis from monkeys to adult humans (Tauraso 1973). One of the difficulties in controlling the disease is that it is difficult to detect the *Shigella* carriers that act as a reservoir of infection.

Epidemiology

Monkeys' hands are invariably contaminated with their own faeces, so continual ano–oral reinfection with the *Shigella* organism will occur. An asymptomatic carrier state can occur when the *Shigella* organisms are carried in, and intermittently shed from, the colonic mucosa. Contact can occur between groups of animals as faecal matter is often splashed when washing down the cages. Natural sterilisation by desiccation and UV light do not occur inside the animal house and flies act as an important vector of the disease. Controlling of flies has been found to reduce the transmission of *Shigella* and decrease the incidence of disease (Cohen *et al.* 1991). This is important in the management of primate facilities as flies are difficult to control in outdoor facilities, and they are often brought inside a building on supplies of fresh fruit and may then spread the disease between individuals. Cockroaches are also a possible vector of the disease if not controlled (Weil *et al.* 1971).

Adequate hygiene and disinfection in the animal house are vital to break the cycle of reinfection. Rooms should be routinely cleaned with a suitable disinfectant (e.g. Virkon 2%). Infected animals should be bathed in a bactericidal shampoo after recovery from enteric illness before being returned to the colony. Adequate protective clothing must be provided for staff and overshoes or disinfectant footbaths must be provided and used correctly. Equipment should not be shared between different rooms or areas.

Sampling method: Frequency of sampling

One problem with diagnosis of *Shigella* is that the average detection rate in clinical cases is only 44% (Lindsey *et al.* 1971). The detection of *Shigella* infection is variable and single samples are not sufficiently reliable to state that an animal is free from infection. If the detection rate is 44% on any one sample, then by sampling on 3 consecutive days, the probability of detecting infection rises to 82% ($P = 1 - (1 - x)^n$ where $x =$ detection rate, $n =$ number of days sampled.) This probability rises to 90% for 4 days of sampling and 94.5% for 5 days of sampling. A compromise has to be reached between the probability of detecting infection, the costs of laboratory examinations and the ability of any in-house laboratory, in terms of equipment and staff, to handle large numbers of samples on consecutive days. The common practice is to screen animals on 3 consecutive days, and this is repeated three times. All clinical cases of diarrhoea should also be sampled on 3 consecutive days. Samples should be taken for 3 consecutive days 1 week after arrival in a new unit, and 1 week after any period of stress when they are more likely to be shedding *Shigella* if they are present (e.g. after surgery). Random sampling should also be carried out on a regular basis. The microbiologist should select cage/area numbers from a table of random numbers and samples are then sent in to the laboratory for 3 consecutive days. Juvenile animals should be sampled in the immediate post-weaning period, also for 3 days, when they are likely to be maximally stressed.

Sampling method: Collection and transport of samples

In sampling human patients to screen for the presence of *Shigella* infection, rectal swabs or faecal samples may be examined. When dealing with non-human primates the taking of adequate rectal swabs may necessitate tranquilisation of the animal, rendering it an unsuitable method for mass screening of some monkey populations of larger species. In these cases, faecal samples are usually examined, as fresh a sample as possible being selected. If animals are kept in groups, as many samples as there are animals in the area are collected, with each sample being collected from different faecal masses. A significant factor in reducing the detection rate of *Shigella* is the transport time of the sample from the monkey to the laboratory. Ideally, direct plate the sample for maximal recovery of *Shigella* or, if there must be a delay, then use transport media. The most satisfactory method for transportation of the samples is in phosphate-buffered saline at 4°C (Shimoda *et al.* 1991).

Sampling method: Microbiological detection

Intracellular maintenance of *Shigella* in carriers will decrease the incidence of detection and attempts at culture during acute shigellosis may also be unrewarding (Lindsey *et al.* 1971) since, the more blood that is present in the sample, the less likely an isolate will be found (Bourne, 1975). Other reasons for cases of *Shigella* going unrecognised or undetected are that some selective and differential media traditionally employed in the examination of faecal samples for enteric pathogens have been found to be too inhibitory for the *Shigella* organisms. The choice of enrichments and primary plating media is very important for the recovery of *Shigella*. Traditional cultural methods assumed that the conditions for isolation of *Salmonella* would also be conducive to the growth of *Shigella*, but *Shigella* is closely related to the genus *Escherichia*, which the highly selective media were designed to inhibit. Therefore a combination of different selective media should be employed to allow optimal recovery of *Shigella*.

Pathogenesis

The *Shigella* bacterium colonises the intestine and invades the mucosal epithelial cells by bacteria-induced phagocytosis. The bacteria then multiply intracellularly, the infectious focus enlarges, the goblet cells empty and mucosal erosion and ulceration develop resulting in the passage of mucoid and bloody stools (Rout *et al.* 1975).

Treatment

In human medicine it is considered that the greater the use of antibiotics, the more likely resistance is to develop (Ceyhan *et al.* 1988), and antibiotics are avoided for the treatment of diarrhoea. However in monkeys, the prompt administration of the most efficient antimicrobial agent based on *in vitro* sensitivity tests, together with measures to control emaciation and dehydration, contribute to a significant reduction in mortality from enteric infections (Arya *et al.* 1973). A short course of suitable antibiotic at an adequate dose should be given where necessary. It is important to monitor the changes in antibiotic resistance of the bacteria and adjust the treatment accordingly. There must also be constant attention paid to the possibility of concomitant disease processes and these must be diagnosed and treated accordingly. Severely ill animals must be treated individually. Ideally these severely affected animals should be removed to separate facilities for this additional treatment and the contaminated area should be sterilised and the animal only returned after it has been bathed in surgical scrubs to clean the coat. Fluids by intravenous infusion are used to treat these individual severe cases, spasmolytics and analgesics may be used to control abdominal discomfort and corticosteroids are used to control chronic colitis, which may be a potential sequela. On recovery, live yogurt may be fed to help recolonise the gut bacteria to reduce the occurrence of colitis.

All cases of diarrhoea should be sampled to monitor the bacteriological status of the colony and, if the infection is widespread, the colony should be isolated and treated. It is vitally important to dose the animals with a suitable antibiotic at an adequate dose and for an adequate length of time. Treatment will not immediately eliminate the carrier state but simply reduces the number of bacilli below a level at which they can be detected (Good *et al.* 1969). As numbers are reduced to undetectable levels, so the incidence of disease will be markedly reduced, but there may still be occasional clinical cases or bacterial isolations. However these can rapidly be contained.

Eradication will depend on a prolonged programme of breaking the cycles of infection and transmission by improving hygiene and detecting and treating carriers (Wolfensohn 1998). In some units the presence of *Shigella* is accepted, since, with good husbandry, control is possible even with healthy carriers in the colony, provided the animals are not subjected to undue levels of stress which may precipitate clinical disease. However given the zoonotic potential, consideration must then be given to the assessment of risk to staff and since the secondary complications possible from the type of pathology induced by shigellosis could be numerous and serious, it is important to keep animals free from disease wherever possible.

Parasitic infections

There are many enteric parasitic infections of primates, many are non-pathogenic, some are zoonotic, a few require diagnosis and treatment. Full details may be found in Owen (1992). The important ones to consider are the protozoans *Giardia* spp., *Trichomonas* spp., *Entamoeba histolytica*, *Cryptosporidium* spp., *Balantidium* spp., and the metazoans *Strongyloides* spp. and *Trichuris* spp.

The protozoa may be treated with agents such as metronidazole and the metazoans with ivermectin.

Melioidosis

This infection, due to *Pseudomonas pseudomallei*, is uncommon but is found occasionally in imported monkeys from the Philippines and Indonesia. Affected animals have abscesses of the spleen and liver and sometimes of the skin and other soft tissues. Diagnosis is by ELISA test to demonstrate the presence of antibodies to the *Ps. pseudomallei*. The clinical manifestations of the disease are very varied and can be fulminant septicaemia with sudden death or just an asymptomatic seroconversion. The organism can remain latent for many years before causing symptoms and so should be on the list of differential diagnoses in any animal from an area where the disease is endemic, irrespective of the period since it was imported. The incidence of melioidosis in endemic areas is seasonal and increases when the rainy season is exceptionally wet. Environmental contamination occurs and can be difficult to reduce, despite the use of disinfectants. The zoonotic risks must be considered particularly in people who may be immunocompromised.

Other diseases

It may be desirable to include other diseases in the health-screening programme, such as *Leptospira* or *Toxoplasma gondii*, depending on individual circumstances. For further information on screening of primate colonies see FELASA Working Group on Non-Human Primate Health (1999).

HUSBANDRY-RELATED DISEASES

A management strategy for dealing with such problems as fight injuries or nutritional imbalances, which may be encountered with increasing use of foraging and group housing, should be developed and built into any primate health-management programme. The benefit of social housing is that the environment is dynamic, unpredictable and variable so there is little habituation, but there are increased risks of infection, wounding and competition for food. With good management strategies these risks can be minimised but not altogether removed.

Fighting injuries

Monkeys live according to strict social rules, and to sort out the transgressors there will inevitably be some fights and some animals will get injured. They may even be killed. It is questionable whether it is better to live in isolation safely, or in a group and run the risk of being beaten up, but for the benefit of the greater good it is widely accepted that monkeys should be kept in groups. In all primate societies, whether human or monkey, there will be the occasional social misfit who will have to be removed either for their own safety or for the benefit of the remainder of that group. It is important to maintain a flexible approach to the management and use of monkey colonies to ensure that such individuals are used to maximum benefit and neither wasted nor left to suffer social deprivation simply because they don't fit in. The size of the group is important, if not more important than the amount of space per animal. Many primate species live naturally in fairly large groups (such as macaques) and while putting a small group of animals or a pair together will give them company, there appears to be a higher incidence of fights and unsettled behaviour in these groups than in larger groups, even if the amount of floor space per monkey is reduced in the latter case.

Treating monkeys with fight injuries

All injured animals should be examined and treated as soon as possible after being wounded to minimise the chances of infection. If given within 6 hours of the wounding, intensive treatment can virtually eliminate infection. A balance must be struck between examining all fight casualties under sedation in a procedures room, or making a judgement on the seriousness just by observing the animal in the cage; remembering that an injured animal will often try to hide the wound, and many wounds may appear superficial while the underlying damage is more serious. Assess the condition of the animal in the cage and give a reduced dose of sedative if the animal's consciousness appears to be depressed. Check the entire animal for lacerations, puncture wounds, bruising and seemingly minor abrasions. Pay particular attention to hands and feet, ears and the tail base. Follow one of the treatment protocols below, but move the animal onto a more intensive protocol if there is any deterioration in its general condition. All animals will require supportive care in the period after examination. Place animals on insulating bedding for examination and recovery, monitor the rectal temperature and use heat pads to maintain body temperature. In severe cases, the animal may be hypothermic on examination and require warmed i.v. fluids in addition to supplementary heating to raise the body temperature. Ensure that adequate analgesia is provided, either using opioids or NSAIDs, as appropriate, in conjunction with any anaesthetic used.

1. Protocol for animals with minor lacerations only, no depression

Under sedation, clip and clean around the wounds. Flush copiously with dilute chlorhexidine, or sterile saline. Apply products such as Dermisol® cream or solution or Intrasite™ gel to minor areas of necrotic tissue. If required, give i.v. antibiotic (e.g. amoxicillin 20 mg/kg, Amoxil® injection), and continue treatment with oral or injectable antibiotic daily for 5 days, as necessary.

2. Protocol for animals with major lacerations and puncture wounds, no depression

Under sedation, clip and clean the wounds. If necessary, induce general anaesthesia via an indwelling i.v. cannula or butterfly needle (cephalic or saphenous vein). Assume puncture wounds have hidden damage beneath the skin and open them up to investigate fully. Flush wounds copiously with sterile saline. Suture torn muscles and subcutaneous tissues with absorbable suture (e.g. Ethicon Vicryl™) and close skin with subcuticular Vicryl™ sutures if possible. Place skin staples as necessary if the wound is fresh. Assess if animals are dehydrated or have lost blood, replace fluids at an appropriate rate i.v. if necessary. If wounds are highly contaminated or not amenable to stitching (second intention healing required) or extra wound support is needed, dress wounds as follows. Monkeys will tolerate bandages very well if they are applied correctly. When dressing limbs include the hand or foot or check to ensure that there has been no swelling distal to the bandage. Continue antibiotic treatments for 5 days or until wounds are healing. Application of dressings:

- 1st layer: Non-stick dressing adjacent to the wound (e.g. Allevyn™ – Smith & Nephew), or a dressing containing anti-microbial agents such as silver or charcoal (e.g. Acticoat™ – Smith & Nephew or Activate™ – Robinson Animal Health Care)
- 2nd layer: Padding layer (e.g. Soffban™), thickness of layer depends on degree of support required
- 3rd layer: Conforming bandage (e.g. Kling™, Vet-band™)
- 4th layer: Outer layer of cohesive (e.g. Co-Form™, Co-Ripwrap™) or adhesive bandage (e.g. Elastoplast®)

Remember to ensure that no fur is stuck to the bandage, causing discomfort. Monkeys will tolerate a comfortable bandage very well but for animals that are very curious an additional, separate piece of the outer layer bandage placed over the top will keep it occupied and away from the principal dressing. Change dressings every 3–4 days.

3. Protocol for animals with multiple small lacerations and/or bruising, and those which appear depressed

These animals may succumb to septicaemia and/or renal failure several days after the injury, and require intensive therapy if they are to survive. If necessary, sedate using a low dose of sedative for examination. Insert an indwelling i.v. cannula, preferably into a cephalic vein. Give i.v. antibiotic (e.g. amoxicillin 20 mg/kg) and corticosteroids (e.g Solu-medrone V™ – Pfizer Ltd, or Dexadreson™ – Intervet UK Ltd). Give i.v. fluids for maintenance (0.9% saline or 0.18% saline with 4% glucose). Warm the fluids first, give 40–80 ml/kg per 24 hours, more if dehydrated, checking hydration status and urination frequently. Do not be tempted to have the fluids running in too fast, since this will result in pulmonary oedema. For example, a 5-kg monkey which is not dehydrated, needs about 5×60 ml (300 ml) fluid/24 hours (12.5 ml/hour, or about 4 drops from a giving set per minute). If the animal develops areas of gangrenous necrosis following injuries, these must be treated intensively. This is often due to *E. coli* infection, and may not be controlled adequately by antibiotics alone. Induce general anaesthesia, surgically debride necrotic areas as much as possible and flush with sterile saline, give intravenous antibiotics, and apply dressings to affected areas. When the animal has recovered from anaesthesia, give flunixin (e.g. Finadyne™ – Schering-Plough Animal Health) s.c. (1 ml per 10 kg) to counteract any toxaemia.

Nutritional problems

Clinical problems may be brought about by the increasing provision of forage mix in addition to normal pelleted diet. Although the forage mixes are all well balanced nutritionally, this assumes that the monkey will not pick out its favourite bits and leave the rest to those animals lower in the social order. By introducing an element of choice, the diet may become unbalanced and problems, such as rickets in juvenile animals, may arise from this. For further information see Chapter 4 on Nutrition.

New World primate colitis

New World primate species suffer from a variety of large-bowel syndromes which may be grouped together. Known variously as marmoset and tamarin colitis, or marmoset wasting syndrome, the condition is multifactorial. Possible causes include inadequate protein in the diet, pathogens such as *Campylobacter* or coronavirus, abnormal bowel flora (dysbiosis), immune mediation or hepatic hemosiderosis. Provision of gluten-free diets may assist in the management of these conditions. Cotton-top tamarins also get colonic adenocarcinoma, it has been postulated that this is due to accumulations of white blood cells and development of microabscesses, leading to dilatation and enterocyte damage with microulcerations that coalesce to form mucosal ulcers. This results in increased mitotic activity with regeneration, mononuclear inflammation, microherniation of glands, dysplasia and in some cases neoplasia. There is evidence in marmosets of fatal lymphoproliferative disease associated with a gamma herpesvirus (Ramer *et al.* 2001), which is the end stage of what is known as marmoset wasting syndrome. The possible association of this novel virus with tumours and chronic enteritis may have implications if these animals are used for research on the immune system.

Post-weaning diarrhoea

Post-weaning chronic diarrhoea is significantly associated with body weight at weaning, rather than being associated with age (Munoz-Zanzi 1999). An episode of pre-weaning diarrhoea is a good predictor for the occurrence of post-weaning diarrhoea, possibly since this may alter the function of intestinal mucosa and thus reduce the absorption of nutrients. This leads to reduced growth, smaller weight, impaired immune function and consequently post-weaning diarrhoea.

SEDATION OF PRIMATES

The following is a selection of drugs that may be used to sedate primates to facilitate handling. For further information consult your veterinary surgeon and see Foster *et al.* (1996) and Sun *et al.* (2003). In the UK, all these drugs are prescription-only medicines and therefore must only be used under veterinary direction.

- *Ketamine* (5–25 mg/kg i.m.) is the drug of choice. Lower doses produce heavy sedation. Higher doses produce light anaesthesia. Peak effect is reached in 5–10 min and lasts 30–60 min.
- *Alphaxalone/Alphadolone* (12–18 mg/kg i.m.) is good for small primates, and produces heavy sedation. Additional doses (6–9 mg/kg i.v.) produce surgical anaesthesia. Peak effect is reached 5 min after i.m. injection and lasts 45 min. For larger primates the volume that has to be injected is too large for it to be used by this route.
- *Acepromazine* (0.2 mg/kg i.m.) produces sedation but insufficient for safe handling.
- *Diazepam* (1 mg/kg i.m.) also produces insufficient sedation for handling of larger primates, but may be used in combination with ketamine.
- *Fentanyl* (0.05–0.1 mg/kg s.c. or i.m.) produces heavy sedation and good analgesia.
- *Medetomidine* can be used to produce moderate sedation which can be reversed with atipamezole. Use medetomidine at 50–100 µg/kg i.m.; reverse with atipamezole at 250–500 µg/kg i.m. Useful in combination with ketamine.
- *Atropine* (0.05 mg/kg i.m.) may be given to reduce bradycardia and salivary secretions, especially when ketamine is used.

Once sedated, the monkey can be examined systematically from head to toe.

FURTHER READING

ACDP (1998) *Working Safely with Simians: Management of Infection Risks.* Advisory Committee on Dangerous Pathogens. The Stationery Office, London.

Arya, S.C., Verghese, A. & Agarwal, D.S. (1973). Shigellosis in rhesus monkeys in quarantine. *Laboratory Animals,* **7,** 101–109.

Bennett, B.T., Abee, C.R. & Hendrickson, R. (eds) (1998) *Nonhuman Primates in Biomedical Research: Diseases.* Academic Press, San Diego, California.

Boulter, E.A., Kaler, S.S., Heberling, R.L., Guarjardo, J.E. & Lester, T.L. (1982) A comparison of neutralization tests for the detection of antibodies to *Herpesvirus simiae* (monkey B virus). *Laboratory Animal Science*, **32** (2), 150–152.

Bourne, G.H. (1975) *The Rhesus Monkey*. Academic Press, London.

Brack, M. (1996). Gongylonematiasis in the common marmoset (*Callithrix jacchus*). *Laboratory Animal Science*, **46**, 266–270.

Brusasca, P.N., Peters, R.L., Motzel, S.L., *et al.* (2003) Antigen recognition by serum antibodies in non-human primates experimentally infected with *Mycobacterium tuberculosis*. *Comparative Medicine*, **53**, 165–172.

Centers for Disease Control and Prevention (1997) Non-human primate spumavirus infections among persons with occupational exposure. *Morbidity and Mortality Weekly Report*, **46**, 6.

Ceyhan, M., Dilmen, U. & Korten, V. (1988) *Shigella* diarrhoea and treatment. *Lancet*, **332** (8061), 45–46.

Chellman, G.J., Lukas, V.S., Eugui, E.M., *et al.* (1992) Activation of B virus (*Herpersvirus simiae*) in chronically immunosuppressed cynomolgus monkeys. *Laboratory Animal Science*, **42**, 146–151.

Cohen, D., Green, M. & Block, C. (1991) Reduction of transmission of shigellosis by control of house flies (*Musca domestica*). *Lancet*, **337**, 993.

Eberle, R. & Hilliard, J.K. (1995) The simian herpesviruses. *Infectious Agents and Disease*, **4**, 55–70.

FELASA [Federation of Laboratory Animal Science Associations] Working Group on Non-Human Primate Health (Weber, H., Berge, E., Finch, J., *et al.* (1999) Health monitoring of non-human primate colonies. *Laboratory Animals*, **33** (Suppl. 1), S1:3–S1:18.

Foster, A., Zeller, W. & Pfannkuche, H-J. (1996) Effect of thiopental, saffan and propofol anaesthesia on cardiovascular parameters and bronchial smooth muscle in the rhesus monkey. *Laboratory Animal Science* **46**, 327–334.

Fowler, M.E. (ed.) (1978, 1986, 1993) *Diseases of Zoo and Wild Animals*, 1st–3rd edns. W.B. Saunders, USA.

Good, R.C., May, B.D. & Kawatomari, T. (1969) Enteric pathogens in monkeys. *Journal of Bacteriology*, **97**, 1048–1055.

Hilliard, J.K. & Ward, J.A. (1999) B-virus-specific pathogen-free breeding colonies of macaques (*Macaca mulatta*): retrospective study of seven years of testing. *Laboratory Animal Science*, **49**, 144–148.

Honess P., Johnson P. & Wolfensohn S. (2004) A study of behavioural responses of non-human primates to air transport and re-housing. *Laboratory Animals*, **38**, 119–132.

Holmes, G.P., Chapman, L.E., Stewart, J.A., *et al.* and the B virus working group (1995) Guidelines for the prevention and treatment of B-virus infections in exposed persons. *Clinical Infectious Diseases*, **20**, 421–439.

ILAR (1976) Long term holding of laboratory rodents. *Institute of Laboratory Animal Resources News*, **19**, 1–25.

Kalter, S.S., Heberling, R.L., Cooke, A.W., *et al.* (1997) Viral infections of nonhuman primates: Overview of data from Viral Reference Laboratory San Antonio on results from 53,000 tests. *Laboratory Animal Science*, **47**, 461–467.

Kanaujia, G.V., Garcia, M.A., Bouley, D.M., *et al.* (2003) Detection of early secretory antigenic target-6 antibody for diagnosis of tuberculosis in non-human primates. *Comparative Medicine*, **53**, 602–606.

Kennedy, F.M., Astbury, J. & Needham, J. R. (1992) Shigellosis due to occupational contact with non-human primates. *Epidemiology and Infection*, **110**, 247–254.

Kobune, F., Takahashi, H., Terao, K., *et al.* (1996) Non-human primate models of measles. *Laboratory Animal Science*, **46**, 315–320.

Lerche, N.W., Cotterman, R.F., Dobson, M.D., *et al.* (1997) Screening for simian type D retrovirus infection in macaques, using nested polymerase chain reaction. *Laboratory Animal Science*, **47**, 263–268.

Lindsey, J.R., Hardy, P.H. & Baker, H.J. (1971) Observations on shigellosis and development of multiple resistant *Shigellas* in *Macaca mulatta*. *Laboratory Animal Science*, **21**, 832–844.

MAFF (1994) *Condition Scoring of Sheep: Action on Animal Welfare*. Ministry of Agriculture, Fisheries & Food (MAFF) Publications, London.

Munoz-Zanzi, C.A., Thurmond, M.C., Hird, D.W. & Lerch, N.W. (1999) Effect of weaning time and associated management practices on postweaning chronic diarrhoea in captive rhesus monkeys (*Macaca mulatta*). *Laboratory Animal Science*, **49**, 617–621.

Norcott, J.P. & Brown, D.W. (1993) Competitive radioimmunoassay to detect antibodies to herpes B virus and SA8 virus. *Journal of Clinical Microbiology*, **31**, 931–935.

O'Sullivan, M.G., Anderson, D.K., Lund, J.E., *et al.* (1996) Clinical and epidemiological features of simian parvovirus infection in cynomolgus macaques with severe anaemia. *Laboratory Animal Science*, **46**, 291–297.

Owen, D.G. (1992) *Parasites of Laboratory Animals*. Laboratory Animal Handbooks No. 12. Royal Society of Medicine Press, London.

Preston, R. (1994) *The Hot Zone*. Doubleday, London.

Price, R.E., Leeds, N.E., Hazle, J.D., *et al.* (1997) Magnetic resonance imaging of the central nervous system of the rhesus monkey. *Laboratory Animal Science*, **47**, 304–312.

Ramer, J.C., Florence, D., Garber, R.L., *et al.* (2001) Fatal lymphoproliferative disease associated with a novel gamma herpesvirus in a captive population of common marmosets. Paper given at *American Society of Primatologists 2001 Meeting*, Wisconsin Regional Primate Research Center, University of Wisconsin, Madison.

Rout, W.R., Formal, S.B. & Giannella, R.A. (1975) Pathophysiology of *Shigella* diarrhoea in the rhesus monkey: Intestinal transport, morphological and bacteriological studies. *Gastroenterology*, **68**, 270–278.

Schou, S. & Hansen, A.K. (2000) Marburg and Ebola virus infections in laboratory non-human primates: A literature review. *Comparative Medicine*, **50**, 108–123.

Shimoda, K., Maejima, K. & Kuhara, T. (1991) Stability of pathogenic bacteria from laboratory animals in various transport media. *Laboratory Animals*, **25**, 228–231.

Slomka, M.J., Brown, D.W., Clewley, J.P., *et al.* (1993) Polymerase Chain Reaction for detection of herpesvirus simiae (B virus) in clinical specimens. *Archives of Virology*, **131**, (1–2), 89–99.

Sun, F.J., Wright, D.E. & Pinson, D.M. (2003) Comparison of ketamine versus combination of ketamine and medetomidine in injectable anaesthetic protocols: chemical immobilization in macaques and tissue reaction in rats. *Contemporary Topics*, **42**, 32–37.

Tauraso, N.M. (1973) Review of recent epizootics in nonhuman primate colonies and their relation to man. *Laboratory Animal Science*, **23**, 201–210.

Vogel, P., Weigler, B.J., Kerr, H., *et al.* (1994) Seroepidemiologic studies of cytomegalovirus infection in a breeding population of rhesus macaques. *Laboratory Animal Science*, **44**, 25–30.

Ward, J.A. & Hilliard, J.K. (2002) Herpes B-virus-specific pathogen-free breeding colonies of macaques: serologic test results and the B-virus status of the macaque. *Contemporary Topics in Laboratory Animal Science*, **41**, 36–41.

Ward, J.A. & Hilliard, J.K. (1994) B-Virus-specific pathogen-free breeding colonies of macaques: Issues, surveillance and results in 1992. *Laboratory Animal Science*, **44**, 222–228.

Weigler, B.J. (1992) Biology of B-virus in macaque and human hosts: A review. *Clinical Infectious Disease*, **14**, 555–567.

Weigler, B.J., Hird, D.W. & Hilliard, J.K. (1993) Epidemiology of cercopithecine herpesvirus 1 infection and shedding in a large breeding cohort of rhesus macaques. *Journal of Infectious Diseases*, **167**, 257–263.

Weigler, B.J., Scinicarello, F. & Hilliard, J.K. (1995) Risk of venereal B virus (Cercopithecine Herpesvirus 1) transmission in rhesus monkeys using molecular epidemiology. *Journal of Infectious Diseases*, **171**, 1139–1143.

Weil, J.D., Ward, M.K. & Spertzel, R.O. (1971) Incidence of *Shigella* in conditioned rhesus monkeys (*Macaca mulatta*). *Laboratory Animal Science*, **21**, 434–437.

Weir, E., Bhatt, P.N., Jacoby, R.O., et al. (1993) Infrequent shedding and transmission of herpesvirus simiae from seropositive macaques. *Laboratory Animal Science*, **43**, 541–544.

Whitley, R.J. (1990) Cercopithecine herpesvirus I (B virus). In: *Virology* (eds B.N. Fields and D.M. Knipe), pp. 2063–2075. 2nd edn. Raven Press, New York.

Wolfensohn, S.E. (1998) *Shigella* infection in macaque colonies: Case report of an eradication and control program. *Laboratory Animal Science*, **48**, 330–333.

Wolfensohn, S.E. & Gopal, R. (2001) Interpretation of serological test results for Simian herpes B virus. *Laboratory Animals*, **35**, 315–320.

Wolfensohn, S.E. & Lloyd, M.H. (2003) *Handbook of Laboratory Animal Management and Welfare*, 3rd edn. Blackwell Science, Oxford.

Zwartouw, H.T., Macarthur, J.A., Boulter, E.A., et al. (1984) Transmission of B-virus infection between monkeys especially in relation to breeding colonies. *Laboratory Animals*, **18**, 125–130.

Table 5.1 Useful data, marmoset.

Biological data		Breeding data	
Adult weight (grams)	300–400	Puberty(months)	8
Diploid number	46	Age to breed (years)	1.5–2
Food intake	20 g daily New World monkey pelleted diet	Gestation (days)	140–148 Average 145
		Litter size	Usually dizygotic twins Can be 1–4 offspring
Lifespan (years)	10–16	Birthweight (grams)	25–35
Rectal temperature (°C)*		Weaning age[†]	6 weeks to 6 months
Day	38.6		
Night	36.3		
Heart rate/min*	230–312	Oestrous cycle (days)	14–28. Few overt signs of oestrus
Mean arterial pressure (mmHg)*		Comments	
Day	65–100		Interbirth interval
Night	50–95		154–178 days
Blood volume (ml/kg)	70		
Haematological data		**Biochemical data**	
RBC ($\times 10^6$/mm^3)	5.7–6.95	Serum protein (g/dl)	6.6–7.1
PCV (%)	45–52	Albumin (g/dl)	3.8
Hb (g/dl)	14.9–17	Globulin (g/dl)	2.7–3.9
WBC ($\times 10^3$/mm^3)	7.3–12.8	Glucose (mg/dl)	126–228

Table 5.1 (Continued).

Haematological data		Biochemical data	
Neutrophils (%)	26–62	Blood urea nitrogen (mg/dl)	51.8
Lymphocytes (%)	30–67	Creatinine (mg/dl)	0.9–1.2
Eosinophils (%)	0.6–4.2	Total bilirubin (mg/dl)	0.4–0.6
Monocytes (%)	0.4–5		
Basophils (%)	0.1–1.1		
Platelets ($\times10^3$/mm^3)	490		

* Marked diurnal changes: heart rate, arterial pressure, activity and body temperature all fall at night.
† Young can suckle for longer, particularly if stressed.

Table 5.2 Useful data, squirrel monkey.

Biological data		Breeding data	
Adult weight (grams)		Puberty(years)	
Male	550–1100	Male	3.5
Female	350–750	Female	1.5
Diploid number	44	Age to breed (years)	
		Male	3.5
		Female	2.5–3.5
Food intake (grams)	45–60 daily	Gestation (days)	145–150
		Litter size	1
Lifespan (years)	10	Birthweight (grams)	100
Rectal temperature (°C)	39.7	Oestrous cycle (days)	7–13
Heart rate/min	215–265	Comments	Seasonal polyoestrus. Mating March to May
Blood pressure systole (mmHg)	127–160		
Blood pressure diastole (mmHg)	77–83		
Respiratory rate/min	55–70		
Tidal volume (ml)	7.5–8.9		

Haematological data		Biochemical data	
RBC ($\times10^6$/mm^3)	7.5	Serum protein (g/dl)	6.6–7.8
PCV (%)	42	Albumin (g/dl)	4.9–6.3
Hb (g/dl)	14.1	Globulin (g/dl)	3.16
WBC ($\times10^3$/mm^3)	8.0	Glucose (mg/dl)	57–91
Neutrophils (%)	51	Blood urea nitrogen (mg/dl)	25.6–38.4
Lymphocytes (%)	41	Total bilirubin (mg/dl)	0.2
Eosinophils (%)	5	Cholesterol (mg/dl)	199.1
Monocytes (%)	3		
Basophils (%)	<1		

Table 5.3   Useful data, macaques.

Biological data	Rhesus macaque (*Macaca mulatta*)	Cynomolgus macaque (*Macaca fascicularis*)
Adult weight (kg)		
Male	6–11	4–8
Female	4–9	2–6
Diploid number	42	42
Food intake	420 J/kg for maintenance, 525–630 J/kg for production, 840 J/kg for neonates	
Lifespan (years)	20–30	15–25
Temperature (°C)	36–40	37–40
Heart rate/min	120–180*	240
Blood pressure systole (mmHg)	125	As rhesus
Blood pressure diastole (mmHg)	75	As rhesus
Blood volume (ml/kg)	55–80	50–96
Respiratory rate/min	32–50*	

Breeding data

Age at puberty (years)	Male 3–4, female 2–3	3–4
Age to breed (years)	Male 4–5, female 3–5	4–5
Gestation (days)	146–180 Average 164	153–179 Average 167
Litter size	1	1
Birthweight (kg)	0.4–0.55	0.33–0.35
Weaning age (months)	7–14 Can hand rear from birth	14–18
Breeding cycle	Menstrual cycle 28 days	Menstrual cycle 31 days
Comments	Seasonal breeding September to January[†]	Non-seasonal breeding

Haematological data		Biochemical data	
RBC ($\times 10^6$/mm^3)	3.56–6.95	Serum protein (g/dl)	4.9–9.3
PCV (%)	26–48	Albumin (g/dl)	2.8–5.2
Hb (g/dl)	8.8–16.5	Globulin (g/dl)	1.2–5.8
WBC ($\times 10^3$/mm^3)	2.5–26.7	Glucose (mg/dl)	46–178
Neutrophils (%)	5–88	Blood urea nitrogen (mg/dl)	8–40
Lymphocytes (%)	8–92	Creatinine (mg/dl)	0.1–2.8
Eosinophils (%)	0–14	Total bilirubin (mg/dl)	0.1–2
Monocytes (%)	0–11	Cholesterol (mg/dl)	108–263
Basophils (%)	0–6		
Platelets ($\times 10^3$/mm^3)	109–597		

* Values determined under sedation.

† Northen hemisphere.

Table 5.4 Useful data, baboon.

Biological data		Breeding data	
Adult weight (kg)		Puberty (years)	2.5–3
Male	22–30		
Female	11–15		
Diploid number	42	Age to breed male (years)	4.5–5
Lifespan (years)	up to 28	Age to breed female (years)	3.5–4
Rectal temperature (°C)	36–39	Gestation (days)	164–186
			Average 170
Heart rate/min	74–200	Litter size	1
Blood pressure systole (mmHg)	135	Birthweight (kg)	0.87–0.94
Blood pressure diastole (mmHg)	80	Weaning age (months)	5–8
Blood volume (ml/kg)	62–65	Breeding cycle	Menstrual cycle 36 days
Respiratory rate/min	29	Comments	Non-seasonal breeding

Haematological data		Biochemical data	
RBC ($\times 10^6$/mm^3)	4.8	Serum protein (g/dl)	6.6
PCV (%)	35–40	Albumin (g/dl)	3.8
Hb (g/dl)	11.9–12.7	Globulin (g/dl)	2.8
WBC ($\times 10^3$/mm^3)	7.5–9.6	Glucose (mg/dl)	95.9
Neutrophils (%)	51	Blood urea nitrogen (mg/dl)	12
Lymphocytes (%)	43	Creatinine (mg/dl)	1.28
Eosinophils (%)	3	Total bilirubin (mg/dl)	0.33
Monocytes (%)	2–8		
Basophils (%)	0.2		

Chapter 6
Psychological well-being

STRATEGY FOR PSYCHOLOGICAL WELL-BEING

Whatever the type of facility, a written strategy to improve animal well-being will assist in the development of a planned and systematic approach to such things as methods of husbandry and provision of environmental enrichment. This should be developed without losing sight of the *raison d'être* for the facility whether it is for medical or zoological research. The goals of the facility will fall into one or more of the following categories:

- research
- breeding
- sales
- education
- exhibition
- other.

The aims of the well-being programme are:

1. to provide the opportunity for expression of a broad range of species-typical behaviours
2. to provide cognitive stimulation
3. to reduce the incidence of stereotypic and/or self-injurious behaviour
4. to provide predictability of routine procedures and events
5. to provide the opportunity for the animal to alter its environment
6. to train staff and animals for routine husbandry and research procedures.

Plans should be developed to cover specific sections such as social interaction, the methodology of record keeping and environmental enrichment.

Social interaction

A planned development of social interaction will address the different categories of animals and how they will each be dealt with. Firstly, singly housed animals will have a plan for integration, starting with olfactory, auditory and tactile contact then leading on to intermittent company; initially supervised. The plan will then address the interaction for paired animals and groups of animals. Finally, as appropriate, the plan will address the social interaction of the animals with care staff both for routine husbandry as well as other procedures.

Records

Adequate record keeping forms a critical part of the plan, not only to aid its implementation but also to provide an audit trail of compliance and demonstration of improvements in well-being of the animals. The following information on individuals should be kept:

- source
- rearing history
- housing history
- peer group history
- health and behaviour records
- other relevant information.

Monitoring should take place *every* day, it is important to note changes as well as absolute signs in such parameters as: activity, physical signs, menstrual cycles in females, responses to routine husbandry, responses to training and any signs of distress. For additional information on dealing with animals showing behavioural abnormalities see Chapters 5 and 7.

ENVIRONMENTAL ENRICHMENT

Primates have active enquiring minds and fingers and this is accentuated in species that are extractive foragers and generalists, such as macaques. This means that primates are particularly prone to suffering from boredom when placed in a barren, unstimulating environment. Conversely, captive primates can benefit significantly and respond well to efforts to enrich their environment, provided that the enrichment presented to them is appropriate for that species, its ecology and behaviour (Röder & Timmermans 2002). Attempts to enrich the environment of primates will only succeed beyond the short term if the programme of enrichment is continually evolving, presenting constantly novel, appropriate and stimulating challenges to the animals, otherwise boredom will re-emerge. An excellent overview of the reaction of primates to changes in their environment can be seen in Box (1991).

It is important when embarking on an environmental enrichment plan that it is formalised and systematic. An essential part of this is to have a programme of evaluation including the measurement of the effect on the animal: how does it affect the range and frequency of behaviours (including the reduction of undesirable behaviours such as stereotypies and self-harming); how much time is spent interacting with the introduced enrichment; and how both interest and effect may degrade over time (Reinhardt 1990; Hienz *et al.* 1998). Additionally, those (usually animal care staff) responsible for developing enrichment programmes should ensure that the programme is structured and reduces *ad hoc* enrichment. They should consult the literature on the design and success of species-specific enrichment devices, thereby avoid 'reinventing the wheel' and potentially making the same mistakes that others have already learnt from and published. Articles published in *Laboratory Primate Newsletter* (http://www.brown.edu/Research/Primate/enrich. html) and the Animal Welfare Institute's database of 'Environmental Enrichment for Primates' (Reinhardt & Reinhardt 2003) form vital resources in this respect. Also communication between animal care staff at different facilities is vital for the cross-fertilisation of ideas for safe, effective enrichment. More information and guidance on environment enrichment may be found in Young (2003).

Different categories of environmental enrichment should be defined and then ways can be found to provide for each category and individual items rotated to provide novelty and prevent animals becoming bored with the same things. Examples of categories of enrichment are:

- social enrichment
- physical environment enrichment
  - manipulation of items
  - control of the environment
  - locomotion/climbing/jumping opportunities
  - variation in tactile stimulation
- foraging for food
- learning opportunities to obtain reward (see Chapter 7).

Social environment enrichment

The most substantial difference that can be made to the life of an individual primate is in the provision of social enrichment in the form of appropriate conspecifics' company (Reinhardt 2004; Reinhardt *et al.* 1991). Primates are highly social animals and suffer greatly when they are deprived of social contact as the many social deprivation studies have shown (Harlow 1958; Novak and Suomi 1991). The effect is not only seen in the severe consequences demonstrated by the infant deprivation of maternal contact in the classic studies of Harlow *et al.* (1971), but in the vital buffering effect on the individual provided by the presence of conspecifics when subjected to a stressful event (Vogt *et al.* 1981).

Most primates, in the wild or when given the opportunity in captivity, spend a substantial part of their day grooming either themselves or others in their group (Silk 1987). While self-grooming can clearly be seen as utilitarian, helping to maintain a clean coat, remove parasites and attend to damaged skin, the function of grooming or being groomed by others, allogrooming, is more complex. A considerable body of literature exists debating the function of allogrooming in primates with explanations varying from utilitarian functions of grooming areas of the body that it is not possible or easy for the individual to groom itself (Freeland 1981); nutritional explanations; or the use of allogrooming as a social glue, cementing and reconciling relationships within the socially complex phenomenon that is primate social life (Boccia 1983). The promotion of grooming can be a valuable tool in reducing stereotypic behaviour in primates (Lam *et al.* 1991).

It is accepted that under certain research conditions it is not possible to house animals together with conspecifics due to, for example, the study of some infectious diseases or following temperament altering procedures which may make an animal aggressive or behave in an inappropriate manner towards a cage mate.

Where exceptional justification cannot be provided for solitary housing, primates should always be housed in appropriate groups, in adequately sized accommodation. Care must always be taken if pairing or grouping animals to ensure this is done with due attention to the species' natural grouping patterns, the sex and temperament of individuals. The response of the animals to this enrichment should be monitored.

Interaction with staff during routine husbandry activities, habituation to people and training, using genuinely positive reinforcement techniques, to cooperate with husbandry practices and research protocols, offers an additional opportunity to enrich the lives of captive primates (see Chapter 7). Positive interaction with humans can be rewarding for the animals and serve to reduce greatly the stressfulness of routine procedures, both for the staff and the animals. This does, however, require staff to be trained in the necessary skills for positive reinforcement training and a sensitivity towards the animals that enables them to recognise behaviour that indicates that the animal or animals are anxious or stressed and may become aggressive; thereby avoiding incidents that may cause injury to staff or animals and set back the programme of training.

Monkeys are social animals that live in groups in the wild. Deprivation of social relations will cause stress in a very short time (Novak & Suomi 1991). In the wild macaque groups are composed of matrilines (female kin groups) and immigrant males that are unrelated to them. The matrilines have a rank order that is relative to one another such that the immature female of a high-ranking lineage will dominate the adult females from lower-ranking lineages. Patterns of intragroup activities such as grooming will often be kin-biased. Group size in the macaques varies with species and can range from more than 10 to less than 100 (Rowe 1996). The adult sex ratio is female biased, although natal sex ratios are equal, owing to the higher rate of mortality among males from male–male competition and the risks associated with intergroup migration (Dunbar 1987). The number of adult males present depends on the number of females present. Reflecting this complex social structure in a captive environment so that animals do not receive serious fight wounds provides a significant challenge. Primates must be kept in harmonious, compatible groups; contrary to some opinion, two individual animals put together does not constitute this, except in monogamous species. They should not be caged individually without special justification (for example, for specific types of experiment, and this must be taken into account in the cost:benefit analysis for the justification for carrying out the experiment in that way). Different species have different requirements and it is essential that those using and keeping primates should be familiar with the natural history and biology of the particular species and provide conditions that meet their physiological and ethological needs.

To ensure harmonious relations, it is essential that the group composition of primates should be appropriate (Mason 1991). Compatibility, and hence group composition, in terms of the age and sex of its members depends on the species. In creating groups, the natural social structure of the species should be taken into account. In captive conditions, natural age and sex composition may be inappropriate so that modifications to group structure may be required. Protocols should be established for group management and particular care taken when individuals, having been removed from groups, are then replaced. There have been instances where, in an individual's absence, social relations changed and the individual was then subjected to considerable aggression on being returned to the group. A possible solution to this problem is to isolate all members of a group for a short while and then re-form the group when any individuals that needed to be removed are returned.

Species-specific factors relevant to social enrichment

Strepsirhines

Scent marking is very important in many contexts: territory, reproduction, social hierarchy. In some species, which tend to be solitary foragers, it is one of the principal means by which communication occurs (together with vocalisation) and by which breeding activities are coordinated. It is therefore necessary to provide housing that allows scent marking activities and too frequent or too thorough cage cleaning may be detrimental to the animals' welfare, since it is important to maintain the olfactory environment. Reverse lighting conditions are necessary for nocturnal strepsirhine species, as well as for nocturnal haplorhines such as owl monkeys (*Aotus* spp.).

Callitrichids

These species' normal body posture is to sit on a support with the tail hanging down, and to move by climbing, running and jumping. Since they are arboreal they should not be expected to sit on the floor, even if it is covered with litter such as wood chips, so food and water should be available up on the perching levels. Chemical communication by scent marking, from urine and from special scent glands such as in the anogenital region, is vital for sexual and social behaviour. Disposable items of environmental enrichment, such as cardboard boxes, tubes, tissue paper, plastic bottles, are useful since they can easily be replaced when they become too soiled and a proportion of them can be changed in one cage area, leaving the remaining items to maintain the scent. Visual baffles are needed between adjacent cages as callitrichids are very territorial and will show threat displays and aggressive behaviour towards animals in adjacent cages. Scent from one breeding female will contribute to the suppression of ovulation in others in some species (see Chapter 8). Close proximity of another cage of animals can lead to excessive scent marking to delineate the territory, so that there is soiling of the animals' coats. For marmosets (*Callithrix* spp.) and tamarins (*Saguinus* spp.) the most appropriate group is the family consisting of a breeding pair and up to three sets of offspring, since same-sex strangers are incompatible. These species are considered monogamous although there is debate over this. For experimental purposes, to avoid isolating individuals, same-sex siblings can be kept together (Figure 6.1).

Cebids

These are also arboreal, so use the vertical dimension more than the horizontal one and need the housing to provide places to perch comfortably; although they will explore the floor and forage if a suitable substrate is provided. Cebids tend to eat a small amount of food and drop the rest, going back to retrieve it later in the day. Those with prehensile tails, such as spider monkeys, need furnishings that allow the use of the tail and suspensory postures. Cebids do not have ischial calluses and perch using their feet. Suitable structures must be provided or they will develop sore feet from pressure sores. It is better if such structures are made from poor thermal conductors such as wood or PVC rather

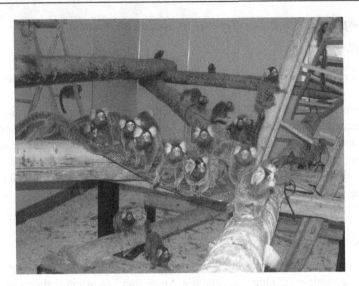

Figure 6.1   Social enrichment for marmosets.

than metal or they can cause hypothermia of the feet. As with the callitrichids, scent is very important in reproductive behaviour, aggressive interactions and other behaviours. Distribution of urine and saliva is important and over-frequent cleaning will disrupt these patterns that are important in social behaviour. Squirrel monkeys (*Saimiri* spp.) can readily be housed in same-sex groups. Efficient breeding requires a minimum of three females and two males, with facilities for males to withdraw out of sight of females to avoid bullying. Capuchins (*Cebus* spp.) have very well developed manipulative abilities. Their busy hands are best directed to destroying disposable items or their attention will be drawn to cage construction and locks!

Circopethicines

Many species of Old World monkeys spend much time on the ground but will flee upwards when startled and will use the perches in the cage differentially, reflecting the social hierarchy. The macaques live naturally in large troops divided into matrilines, whereas the Hamadryas baboons and possibly mandrills and drills live in single male units, although the social groups may comprise several breeding groups. Many African species form mixed species groups in the wild. The high prevalence of simian retro-viruses in African monkeys makes it inadvisable to house mixed groups of Asian and African species since macaques in particular are susceptible to such infections. Different species of macaque will readily hybridise if kept together as a mixed-species pair, but if kept in groups do not tend to do well. Macaques can be housed in same-sex groups, although care should be taken in housing strangers together. Captive breeding is normally in harems with up to 10 females, but groups of 18–28 females with 2 compatible males can also be established. For other species, the advice of appropriate experts should be sought.

Physical environment enrichment

After the provision of suitable space for primates the next most important feature of their physical environment that should be enriched is the furniture. Monkeys are very active animals. In the wild when not foraging for food they will spend much time playing, jumping, swinging and swimming. Enrichment devices need to be designed to provide for these activities. Careful consideration needs to be given to not only the characteristics of the furniture and the material of which it is composed, but also the locomotory and postural behaviour of the species in question.

Primate species vary in the degree to which they are arboreal. Arboreality varies both between major groups, for example all New World primates are exclusively arboreal, and between closely related species; long-tailed macaques (*M. fascicularis*) are more arboreal than their congeneric cousins, the rhesus macaque (*M. mulatta*). For those species that are predominantly or exclusively arboreal it is important that the design of caging and its furniture reflects this. Adding height to caging may create problems when attempting to catch animals, though this can be solved with appropriate training. Perches set at different heights, to allow dominance statement in perching can be supplemented with non-rigid, moving and swinging items that mimic the movement of natural vegetation in the wild (Figure 6.2). Branches, strung old fire hose, ropes, strings of plastic hoops, nets, swinging tyres or barrels have all been used as cage furniture. A barrel will provide visual shelter and serve as swing. Rings set horizontally into the wall at different levels will encourage climbing activity. Swinging inverted cones can act as a food station or a swing. Toys on the ground should give the animal the opportunity to manipulate objects. Tubes made of aluminum or plastic can serve as a shelf and enlarge the surface of the cage. There has been some debate about the use of wood in furniture and toys, but many have found it a valuable and safe material (Primate Enrichment Forum 2000). Use

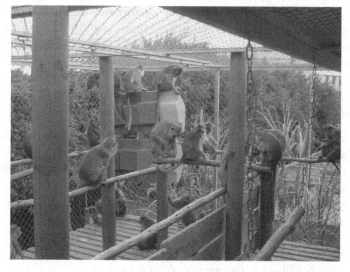

Figure 6.2   Use of perching places.

of rope either alone or as netting has been associated with intestinal obstruction (Eckert 1999) and incidents of strangulation.

While it may be less important to enrich the floor of caging for predominantly arboreal species, for those whose habit is to spend most of their time on the floor care should be taken to provide sufficient terrestrial enrichment. This can be achieved with a selection of small tree 'stumps', balls, barrels as well as foraging toys such as puzzle balls and rubber Kong™ toys filled with frozen fruit juice containing nuts or raisins.

Several macaque species, including the long-tailed and rhesus macaques, are known to be competent swimmers and to enjoy swimming and diving in pools (e.g. for raisins) provided for their enrichment (Anderson *et al.* 1992). Portable or mobile pools made from fibreglass, plastic or tin are therefore a practical and valuable enrichment tool for a range of primate species kept in cages or small enclosures and more permanent water features may be feasible for those in larger areas. It is important, however, that the water is changed frequently enough to avoid it becoming a health risk. Water enrichment of this type may not be appropriate for callitrichids.

There is mixed evidence of the value and effect of enrichment using television, video, music or ambient sounds (e.g. of a forest). Hopkins *et al.* (1989) and Washburn *et al.* (1991) have shown that both chimpanzees and rhesus macaques can learn to play simple computer games. There is also evidence that some primate species will pay attention to television/video enrichment showing, for example, nature films although researchers have mixed views on its enrichment value for chimpanzees, *Pan troglodytes* (Brent & Stone 1996), rhesus macaques, *Macaca mulatta* (Kiyama *et al.* 2003), and vervet monkeys, *Cercopithecus aethiops* (Plesker *et al.* 2001). Music may serve only to distract animals trying to conduct experimental tasks (Carlson *et al.* 1997), but has also been shown to reduce the heart rate of captive baboons (Brent & Weaver 1996) and agitation levels of captive chimpanzees (Howell *et al.* 2003). In humans music has been demonstrated to be valuable in reducing stress in heart patients by drowning out extraneous, potentially distressing noise/sounds (Byers & Smyth 1997). There may be value in presenting video or sound enrichment to captive primates together with the mechanism for them to turn it on or off, and select channels themselves (Harris *et al.* 1999; Howell *et al.* 2003). Primates have been shown to use mirrors to observe activity in adjacent areas (see Figure 6.3).

There are endless opportunities for creative thinking when designing environmental enrichment for primates, much of which can be done very cheaply. The criteria to use when formulating an environmental enrichment programme are:

- Can it seriously injure the animal or the handler?
- Does the animal use it?
- What is the time budget for using it? Items should be rotated so the novelty does not wear off.
- What type of activity is it aimed at, for example feeding, sleeping, jumping, grooming?
- What is the financial cost?
- Is it cleanable or disposable?
- Which animals will use it, for example old or young?

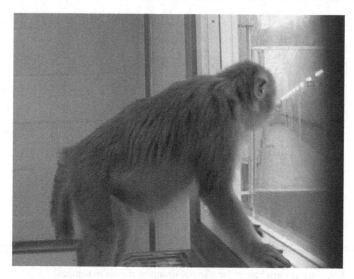

Figure 6.3 Use of a mirror for environmental enrichment.

Feeding-based enrichment

One of the simplest ways of enriching the environment of captive primates is through their diet and their feeding behaviour. In the wild many primate species spend the majority of their day foraging (Oates 1987). It is therefore entirely appropriate to release this normal behaviour in captivity to combat boredom and the development of adverse behaviour. Foraging for food is part of a primate's natural behaviour and is therefore very important in its psychological well-being. It will disperse animals, reduce tension and aggressive interactions, occupy time and reduce stereotypies. The substrate on the enclosure floor should be manipulable and provide comfort as well as being part of the foraging enrichment. Examples of such substrate material are straw, hay, wood wool, shredded paper, sawdust, wood chips, shavings, hemp, soil, bark chippings, and corn cobs (see Figures 2.5 and 6.4).

Successful enrichment programmes make the animal 'work' for food to extend the time taken to process food, since otherwise in captivity the nutrient and energy needs can be fulfilled in a very short time, whereas in the wild it takes about 60% of the animal's daily time budget. Extruded or pelleted diet can be placed in areas that are hard to reach such as in buckets with holes, suspended on chains. Novel foods soon cease to be novel and a continuous programme of change and re-evaluation is required. Treats fed by hand will foster trust and bonding with care staff and provide short-term stimulation but differ greatly from natural foraging.

It is important that programmes of feeding enrichment should be appropriate for the species in question, in the nature of the food provided (fruit, vegetables, gum etc.), the foraging or extraction challenge and the calorific or nutritional contribution to the diet.

Historically many captive primates in research facilities have been kept on grid floors both to simplify cleaning and in some cases for reasons of hygiene. In this instance

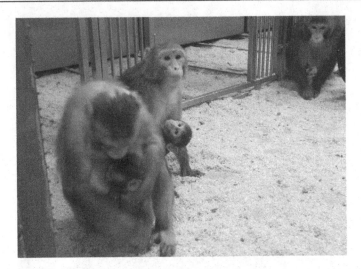

Figure 6.4   Foraging as enrichment for a social group of rhesus macaques.

feeding enrichment can be provided by presenting the animal with fresh fruit or vegetables. While food pellets may provide most of the nutritional requirement of the animal, they make for a monotonous diet. The food should be diverse, not the same dry concentrate diet day after day; the challenge is to provide diversity and yet achieve the correct balance of nutritional components. Food should vary in texture and flavour, for example the addition of banana flavour or cocoa powder to the dry diet will increase palatability (see also Chapter 4). Pellets can be supplemented with a variety of fresh fruit and vegetables; different types of which can be rotated to prevent boredom and predictability.

Captive primates should receive a nutritionally balanced dry food as the principal daily ration, which will also promote oral health. Adding fruit and vegetables will not distort the nutrient balance unless it makes up more than 50% of the diet on a wet-matter basis, since these items are very high in water content. However if fruit and vegetables are fed with a nutritionally balanced component that is also high in water content, such as gel or canned diets, it may be hard for the animal to consume sufficient dry matter to meet its nutrient needs. Dry, very palatable foods, such as nuts and seeds, which are nutritionally incomplete may distort the diet if given in excess, adding vitamin supplements is not satisfactory since this may lead to inadvertent under- or over-dosing.

Sources of protein can also be added, e.g. in the form of thoroughly boiled (to avoid *Salmonella*) eggs, and some primate species (e.g. callitrichids) may benefit from being presented with invertebrates. Live prey provides unpredictability and good foraging opportunities. Examples are invertebrates such as mealworms, wax moth larvae and crickets, which should be fed on a high calcium diet for 2–3 days before being offered. This does not increase the systemic calcium level in the insect but the residue in its gut, which will be consumed by the primate and supplement the dietary level. It is not sufficient to dust the insect with calcium supplementing powder since this tends to be brushed off and lost. Care however is required since live prey can also be a source of pathogens. The feeding of live vertebrate prey also raises ethical and animal welfare issues. Exudates and gum such as gum arabic and high-fibre browse are suitable feeding enrichments for many species. Water may also be used as an enrichment device in many ways, as described earlier.

A foraging tray, containing a substrate such as fine wood chips and a forage mix, containing food such as peanuts, sunflower and poppy seeds and raisins can occupy the animals for considerable periods (Spector *et al.* 1994) (Figure 6.5). Artificial turf has also proved successful as a forage substrate for concealing small food items, and has the advantage of not being particulate and potentially clogging up cage flush-down systems (Bayne *et al.* 1992). A range of puzzle feeders and other general food presentation mechanisms have been developed and these are reviewed by Röder and Timmermans (2002) and Reinhardt (1993).

Different primate species use different foraging techniques, some use hands or tools, some are largely terrestrial while others are largely arboreal. They have different relative cognitive abilities and manual dexterity and these differences need to be accounted for in designing

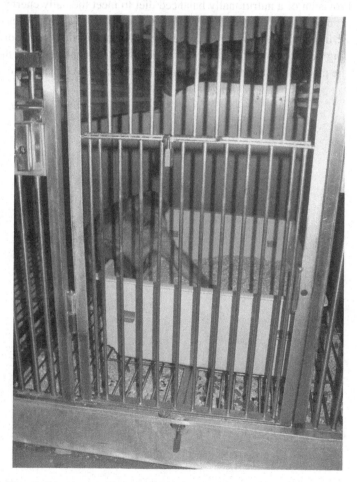

Figure 6.5 Use of a foraging tray over a grid floor.

the feeding programme, if it is to provide environmental enrichment and nutrition successfully. Foraging opportunities can be provided in both time and space. Food should be placed in multiple locations to reduce aggressive monopolisation of a single food source. There is a wide variety of foraging devices on the market, not all are effective in a given situation; different species, ages and individuals prefer different types, so assessment and review are a critical part of the programme. Examples of successful designs of feeding enrichment devices that elicit highly specialised feeding behaviour in certain species are gum feeders for marmosets (McGrew *et al.* 1986) and a simulated 'termite-fishing' device for chimpanzees (Maki *et al.* 1989). The gum feeder is a very simple, cheap device which encourages the natural behaviour of gouging trees to stimulate the production of gum. The animal gouges wood that has holes drilled in it, which are filled with gum Arabic (Figure 6.6). This device has been demonstrated to be successful in reducing stereotypic behaviour and inactivity in common marmosets (*Callithrix j. jacchus*) (Roberts *et al.* 1999).

There is a well-established relationship between nutritional status and susceptibility to disease. Provision of a nutritionally balanced diet to meet the daily energy need and nutrient needs must not be subverted by well-intentioned but ill-advised uses of food in systems of environmental enrichment. It requires knowledge of the science of nutrition, and the feeding behaviour of the species. It is necessary to consider both the physiological and the psychological needs of the animal and to achieve a harmonious balance of the two.

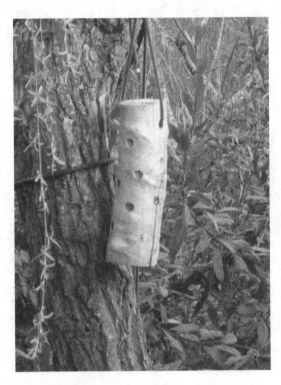

Figure 6.6   A gum feeder for marmosets.

ASSESSMENT OF PSYCHOLOGICAL HEALTH

Despite considerable debate, there is not yet a specific measurement of psychological well-being of primates, but four components can be considered together to build up a picture of the psychological condition of the animal. These are:

1. The physical health of the animal (see Chapter 5).
2. The behavioural repertoire of the animal. It is necessary here to differentiate between normal behaviour and that which is normally seen, which may be abnormal.
3. An objective assessment of the stress the animal is under to determine whether or not it is chronically distressed.
4. An assessment of the animal's coping skills when presented with an environmental challenge or novel stimulus. This will evaluate if it is inquisitive and explorative or if it reverts to an abnormal response and if so, how long it takes to return to baseline level. This will give an indication of the animal's resilience.

It can be seen that none of these parameters alone will give a clear picture of the animal's psychological well-being. A singly housed animal may well be in excellent physical health because it is not exposed to the risk of infections or injury from other animals, there is no competition for food, and no chance of wounding by companions. It will not be trying to maintain its position in a social hierarchy and so may well be less stressed. However such animals frequently show a poor behavioural repertoire with abnormal and even self-harming behaviours and do not have well-developed coping skills. Conversely the benefit of social housing, with the social buffering that this provides, is that the environment is dynamic, unpredictable and variable so there is little habituation, but there are increased risks of infection, wounding and competition for food. With good management strategies these risks can be minimised but not altogether removed.

Sociophysiological information that will aid the determination of well-being will include a knowledge of the background activity of the stress response system, which determines a species' tendency to be an energy consumer or an energy conserver. Measures such as basal metabolic rate, spontaneous feeding patterns, and activity levels will help with this determination. Neuroendocrine responses to routine procedural interventions and rates of habituation to these procedures will identify those procedures that induce large and variant responses. This will assist with planning the most appropriate treatment regime for sick animals. Moving a sick animal to a hospital area may not produce responses that maximise recovery.

Companionship will promote psychological well-being but social living must be viewed as a component of psychological well-being, not as synonymous with it. It depends to some extent whether the monkey is a high-ranking, or a low-ranking individual. Even long-term cage mates may have periods of social instability, but primates have mechanisms for conflict resolution and in a compatible pair one member will be subordinate. This does not mean it is picked on or harassed and does not mean deprivation; it is simply a mutually beneficial means to resolve conflict and reduces the likelihood of injury from physical aggression. Once the animals are in social groups the problems of disease transmission diminish since they are unlikely to be sources of new pathogens for each other. Although social contact is desirable, and having two reasonably compatible animals confined in a cage together may be better than each animal being alone, there need to be other forms of enrichment if boredom and bickering are not to start. The internal furnishings of the cage are vital in this setting (see Chapter 2). Social factors play a role in the aetiology of disease, such as the development of atherosclerosis, which depends not just on diet but also on social ranking and stability (Kaplan *et al.* 1991).

Behavioural modification

See also Chapter 7 on training and modification of behaviour.

As units move away from single caging of monkeys and into better environmental enrichment and improving the welfare of the animals, the stereotypic behaviour patterns, which were once seen so commonly in any laboratory monkey house and in some zoos, have been much reduced. The incidence of self-mutilation is also lower. However it will still be seen occasionally, perhaps in older 'untreatable' animals, which earlier in their lives were kept in sub-standard conditions. The first line of treatment is to improve the environment, but occasionally there will still be individuals that require treatment to control their stress-related behaviour patterns. Just as in humans there are those who cannot cope with everyday life, so this is true with some non-human primate individuals.

The number of animals in satisfactory condition in the facility should be noted and records kept of successful and unsuccessful attempts to modify behaviour.

Specific strategies should be outlined for the following groups:

- aggressive animals
- animals showing stereotypic or self-injurious behaviour
- animals requiring veterinary treatments
- infants under hand rearing
- infants under extra supervision
- juveniles
- experimental animals
- old animals.

If animals that show atypical behaviour are held, then the reasons for these behaviour patterns should be identified and recorded in order to identify and implement methods to benefit future generations and avoid repetition of these cases. For these individuals, there should be records of the presence, and likely aetiology of the atypical behaviour, any remedial action taken, and any special accommodation provided for the affected animal. For a few individuals drug treatment may be indicated with anxiolytics such as the benzodiazepines, or with guanfacine (Macy *et al.* 2000).

FURTHER READING

Anderson, J.R., Peignot, P. & Adelbrecht, C. (1992) Task-directed and recreational underwater swimming in captive rhesus monkeys (*Macaca mulatta*). *Laboratory Primate Newsletter*, **31** (4), 1–5.

Bayne, K., Dexter, S., Mainzer, H., *et al.* (1992) The use of artificial turf as a foraging substrate for individually housed rhesus monkeys (*Macaca mulatta*). *Animal Welfare*, **1**, 39–53.

Boccia, M.L. (1983) A functional analysis of social grooming patterns through direct comparison with self-grooming in rhesus monkeys. *International Journal of Primatology*, **4** (4), 399–418.

Box, H.O. (ed.) (1991) *Primate Responses to Environmental Change*. Chapman Hall, New York.

Brent, L. & Stone, A.M. (1996) Long-term use of television, balls, and mirrors as enrichment for paired and singly caged chimpanzees. *American Journal of Primatology*, **39**, 139–145.

Brent, L. & Weaver, D. (1996) The physiological and behavioural effects of radio music on singly housed baboons. *Journal of Medical Primatology*, **25** (5), 370–374.

Byers, J.P. & Smyth, K.A. (1997) Effect of a music intervention on noise annoyance, heart rate, and pressure in cardiac surgery patients. *American Journal of Critical Care*, **6** (3), 183–191.

Carlson, S., Rama, P., Artchakov, D. & Linnankoski, I. (1997) Effects of music and white noise on working memory performance in monkeys. *Neuroreport*, **8** (13), 2853–2856.

Dunbar, R.I.M. (1987) Demography and reproduction. In: *Primate Societies* (eds B.B. Smuts, D.L. Cheney, R.M. Seyfarth, R.W. Wrangham & T.T. Struhsaker), pp. 240–249. Chicago University Press, Chicago, Illinois.

Eckert, K. (1999) Warning: Rope in environmental enrichment. *Laboratory Primate Newsletter*, **38** (4), 3.

Freeland, W.J. (1981) Functional aspects of primate grooming. *Ohio Journal of Science*, **81** (4), 173–177.

Harlow H.F. (1958) The nature of love. *American Psychologist*, **13**, 573–685.

Harlow, H.F., Harlow, M.K. & Suomi, S.J. (1971) From thought to therapy: Lessons from a primate laboratory. *American Scientist*, **59**, 538–549.

Harris, L.D., Briand, E.J., Orth, R. & Galbicka, G. (1999) Assessing the value of television as environmental enrichment for individually housed rhesus monkeys: A behavioral economic approach. *Contemporary Topics in Laboratory Animal Science* **38** (2), 48–53.

Hienz, R.D., Zarcone, T.J., Turkkan, J.S., *et al.* (1998) Measurement of enrichment device use and preference in singly housed baboons. *Laboratory Primate Newsletter*, **37** (3), 6–10.

Hopkins, W.D., Washburn, D.A. & Rumbaugh, D.M. (1989) Note on hand use in the manipulation of joysticks by rhesus macaques (*Macaca mulatta*) and chimpanzees (*Pan troglodytes*). *Journal of Comparative Psychology*, **103** (1), 91–94.

Howell, S. Schwandt, M., Fritz, J., *et al.* (2003) A stereo music system as environmental enrichment for captive chimpanzees. *Lab Animal Europe*, **3** (10), 16–22.

Kaplan J.R., Adams M.R., Clarkson T.B., *et al.* (1991) Social behaviour and gender in biomedical investigations using monkeys: Studies in atherogenesis. *Laboratory Animal Science*, **41**, 334–343.

Kiyama, A., Taylor, A.J., McCarty, J.L. & Wilson, F.A.W. (2003) A video-display approach to environmental enrichment for macaques. *Laboratory Primate Newsletter*, **42** (3), 1–3.

Lam, K., Rupniak, N.M.J. & Iversen, S.D. (1991) Use of a grooming and foraging substrate to reduce cage stereotypies in macaques. *Journal of Medical Primatology*, **20**, 104–109.

McGrew, W.C., Brennan, J.A. & Russell, J. (1986) An artificial 'gum-tree' for marmosets (*Callithrix j. jacchus*). *Zoo Biology*, **5**, 45–50.

Macy J.D., Beattie T.A., Morgenstern S.E. & Arnsten A.F.T. (2000) Use of guanfacine to control self-injurious behaviour in two rhesus macaques (*Macaca mulatta*) and one baboon (*Papio anubis*). *Comparative Medicine*, **50**, 419–425.

Maki, S., Alford, P.L., Bloomsmith, M.A. & Franklin, J. (1989) Food puzzle device simulating termite fishing for captive chimpanzees *(Pan troglodytes)*. *American Journal of Primatology*, Supplement **1**, 71–78.

Mason, W.A. (1991) Effects of social interaction on well-being: developmental aspects. *Laboratory Animal Science*, **41**, 323–328.

Novak, M. A. & Suomi, S.J. (1991) Social interaction in non-human primates: an underlying theme for primate research. *Laboratory Animal Science*, **41**, 308–314.

Oates, J.F. (1987) Food distribution and foraging behaviour. In: *Primate Societies* (eds B.B. Smuts, D.L. Cheney, R.M. Seyfarth, R.W. Wrangham & T.T. Struhsaker), pp. 197–209. Chicago University Press, Chicago, Illinois.

Plesker, R., H-Hle, K. & Herzog, A. (2001) Prima hedrons, puzzle feeders and television as environmental enrichment for captive African Green Monkeys. *Primate Eye*, **74**, 4 (Abstract).

Primate Enrichment Forum (2000) Wooden objects for enrichment: A discussion. *Laboratory Primate Newsletter*, **39** (3), 1–5.

Reinhardt, V. (1990) Time budget of caged rhesus monkeys exposed to a companion, a PVC perch and a piece of wood for an extended time. *American Journal of Primatology*, **20**, 51–56.

Reinhardt, V. (1993) Foraging enrichment for caged macaques: A review. *Laboratory Primate Newsletter*, **32** (4), 1–5.

Reinhardt, V. (2004) Common husbandry-related variables in biomedical research with animals. *Laboratory Animals*, **38**, 213–235.

Reinhardt, V., Houser, D., Eisele, S., *et al.* (1991) Behavioural responses of unrelated rhesus monkey females paired for the purpose of environmental enrichment. *American Journal of Primatology*, **14**, 135–140.

Reinhardt, V. & Reinhardt, A. (2003) *Environmental Enrichment for Primates: Annotated Database on Environmental Enrichment and Refinement of Husbandry for Nonhuman Primates*. Animal Welfare Institute, Washington DC. http://www.awionline.org/lab_animals/biblio/enrich.htm

Roberts, R.L., Roytburd, L.A. & Newman, J.D. (1999) Puzzle feeders and gum feeders as environmental enrichment for common marmosets. *Contemporary Topics in Laboratory Animal Science*, **38** (5), 27–31.

Röder, E.L. & Timmermans, P.J.A. (2002) Housing and care of monkeys and apes in laboratories: adaptations allowing essential species-specific behaviour. *Laboratory Animals*, **36**, 221–242.

Rowe, N. (1996) *A Pictorial Guide to the Living Primates*. Pogonias Press, East Hampton, New York.

Silk, J.B. (1987) Social behaviour in evolutionary perspective. In: *Primate Societies* (eds B.B. Smuts, D.L. Cheney, R.M. Seyfarth, R.W. Wrangham & T.T. Struhsaker), pp. 318–329. Chicago University Press, Chicago, Illinois.

Spector, M.R., Kowalczyk, M.A., Fortman, J.D. & Bennett, B.T. (1994) Design and implementation of a primate foraging tray. *Contemporary Topics in Laboratory Animal Science*, **33**, 54–55.

Vogt, J.L., Coe, C.L. & Levine, S. (1981) Behavioural and adrenocorticoid responsiveness of squirrel monkeys to a live snake: is flight necessarily stressful? *Behavioural and Neural Biology*, **32** (4), 391–405.

Washburn, D.A., Hopkins, W.D. & Rumbaugh, D.M. (1991) Perceived control in rhesus monkeys (*Macaca mulatta*): Enhanced video-task performance. *Journal of Experimental Psychology*, **17** (2), 123–129.

Young, R.J. (2003) *Environmental Enrichment for Captive Animals*. UFAW Animal Welfare Series. Blackwell Science, Oxford.

Chapter 7
Training of primates

WHY TRAIN PRIMATES?

Primates are intelligent animals, phylogenetically closer to humans than other species. Many other species, domesticated over many generations, are trained to cooperate with man in routine husbandry and others are actually used to work for humans, such as sniffer and guide dogs, messenger pigeons, draft horses. The degree of domestication and selective breeding required to utilise the animals in this way varies depending on the use to which they are being put and the species in question, as well as the degree to which the training is for a behaviour to which the animal species is naturally disposed. Primates remain largely untrained, although pig-tailed macaques (*macaca nemestrina*) have been trained to harvest coconuts in South-east Asia, and are generally regarded as wild animals, which is reflected in the common handling practices used to deal with these species. However many colonies, especially those used in research, have been bred in captivity for many generations and the concept of training the animals to cooperate with procedures, including those for basic husbandry routines, is gaining ground.

The positive benefit of working towards a training programme for individual animals will be that the welfare is improved. Good training and cooperation will reduce the need for the use of sedatives and excessive force when restraining and dealing with the animals. There is no doubt that the use of crush backs and nets for catching primates, even if used well (and there is much opportunity for incorrect or negligent use), is stressful for the animal and provides an opportunity for injury. This is turn reduces the willingness with which care staff catch and examine animals, which can further be detrimental to welfare by increasing the time it takes to observe problems or make an accurate diagnosis in the case of illness. The ability to catch and examine an animal easily will be well rewarded.

The training programme to facilitate handling can be split into component parts:

- human–monkey interaction
- modification of behaviour
- training to permit physical contact
- training to facilitate procedures.

How far along this programme progress is made will depend on the use of the animal and its own temperament and background. For conservation programmes where animals are to be returned to the wild or semi-wild state, living independently, there may be a positive disadvantage to encouraging the animal to form any sort of close relationship with humans, unless supplementary feeding is required. However for those that will live in captivity, having animals that will cooperate with human carers will make life much easier for everyone.

The development of human–animal interaction is best started when the animal is an infant. If the parents are not frightened by the presence of humans the infant should not be either. The aim is that the monkey will not be scared, but equally it is important that the monkey should not become overconfident. Primate social structure is determined very closely by rank and it is important that the human carers do not find themselves competing for rank with a monkey as this may lead to aggression in the monkey and staff injury. The aim is that the monkey has a respect for the carer and does not try to fit that individual into the social hierarchy in which it lives.

SOCIALITY AND PSYCHOLOGICAL WELL-BEING IN PRIMATES

Primates are unusual in the extent to which they seek physical proximity to others. In general being social enhances safety as there is improved vigilance in groups, but there is a very low frequency of predatory episodes against primates in the wild so it is unlikely to be simply a protective strategy. The quest for food is the principal activity of the primate in the wild and the food supplies tend to be concentrated in small patches so in fact being social leads to competition for food resources and for every potential mate there will also be rivals. Although the factors that favour primate social life are poorly understood, there is no doubt that it remains a need.

The psychological well-being of non-human primates is vitally important. The United States Animal Welfare Act 1985 requires researchers 'to provide a physical environment adequate to promote the psychological well-being of primates'. The International Primatological Society (IPS) Guidelines (1993) state 'Primates of many species can be trained for sample procedures . . . and such training is advocated wherever possible using positive reinforcement.'

There are individual differences seen in primates (e.g. relaxed versus anxious individuals), both in nature and in the laboratory. Because of the differences, housing animals in groups creates a more socially relevant context in which to study behavioural and physiological processes in the laboratory but it also brings some potential problems that have to be overcome by good management programmes.

There are four recurring themes to discussions on primate sociality:

1. Species and individuals within species vary in their response to environmental conditions. Social housing does not have the same effect on all species and on all individuals.
2. Housing primates in social groups is a more relevant context in which to conduct research.
3. Data can be collected from group-housed animals, for example by remote monitoring, or the individual can be removed from the group temporarily for testing and then returned.
4. If an animal cannot be housed socially, for example, in some cases of infectious disease research; then there are other non-social methods available to assist with the animal's behavioural needs.

A newborn macaque possesses the potential for a range of developmental outcomes; what actually occurs depends on the stimuli that are provided in the early environment. Social deprivation in early life will produce a range of undesirable behaviours, emotional and motivational disturbances and communication deficits. Neurotic monkeys will not breed well and will be aggressive and dangerous cage mates, leading to difficulties for other animals and staff. The best environment for socialising young macaques is a stable unit including adults and young of both sexes. Sociality is central to the survival of primates, they have long developmental periods, ensuring they have the opportunity to learn from older individuals; and are capable of extensive modification of their behaviour as a function of experience.

The concerns about transmission of disease, individuals inflicting traumatic injuries on each other, competition and possible deprivation of food, water, shelter, and the possibility of social housing interfering with research procedures, have to be weighed against the benefits of social housing, or conversely the costs of solitary, or even pair, confinement. The damage to an animal caused by individual housing may not be immediately apparent as the changes in behaviour may at first be very subtle, but long-term there may be self-mutilation and more obvious damage.

Minimal social housing involves just housing the animals in pairs and there is much folklore about the best way to pair animals: adjacent housing, specific types of cage structure or size of cage, one of the pair should be much larger than the other, carry out the pairing out of the sight, smell and hearing of other animals etc. Rhesus monkeys have a reputation for being more aggressive than many other species of monkey but this is largely as a result of their behaviour towards humans rather than their behaviour towards each other and comparative studies do not support the notion that they are in any way hyperaggressive. Conversely the stump-tailed macaque has a reputation for being docile – towards humans – but they can be quite aggressive towards one another. Animals of advanced age tend to be more compatible than those in prime adulthood.

Introduction of a new group member may promote immediate hostility or it may not produce an immediate response, but hostility could be shown later on. If adult males are put together they will fight if there are females present, however an adult male introduced to a group of juveniles will generally not attack or be attacked. Females will join an attack against an adult male, few males will initiate an attack against a female, but the degree of fighting, retreat etc. will also depend on the amount of space available for retreat and flight. Although mixed introductions may not have much difficulty initially, there remains the potential for future aggression and there needs to be a mechanism for reconciliation and socially sanctioned aggression that does not result in injury but allows for establishment of the social hierarchy. The provision of foraging opportunities in an adequate amount of space is a way of offering this socially sanctioned method of establishing and maintaining the hierarchy that does not result in significant wounding and injury (see Figure 6.4).

There are many different methods of introductions: a gradual approach with mirror contact; direct visual, auditory and olfactory contact; fine mesh then coarse mesh for contact followed by brief periods together before being permanently housed together. However there is no proof that these methods are more or less successful than direct transferences, unless the slower procedure is being used as a predictor of fighting rather than as an habituation process. Habituation may lead to increasing animosity as the animals build up a history of aggressive exchanges and exchanges without resolution. When forming new groups the animals can be introduced one at a time, two already familiar groups can be merged or a group of unrelated individuals all put in together. Using a 'neutral' cage, rather than one in which some of the individuals are already established will help to reduce aggressive encounters. As the group grows larger and friendships are formed the animals are more likely to focus on a single intruder, resulting in aggression. When two groups are merged, there are multiple targets to disperse the attacks so no individual is under continued attack. However with the simultaneous introduction of multiple unfamiliar individuals, there is no social organisation and the conflicts will all be between individuals. This method may appear chaotic and disorganised or ever seen like a riot to the inexperienced human observer, but generally there is far less damage in this setting than when single individuals are added to a group. In some circumstances the use of tranquilisers, such as benzodiazepines, may be indicated to assist in reducing aggressive encounters.

Some of the risks can be minimised by examining the life-history patterns of the species in question. For example squirrel monkeys form sexually segregated societies and so same-sex companions are particularly important. Since they are arboreal and will move large distances in natural forest habitat, generous vertical space and visual barriers will minimise the frequency and severity of antagonistic encounters.

The animal's individual experiences will modify its developmental phenomena since it is a dynamic process that produces the final state. For example sucking and clinging, which should be directed towards the mother, may become directed towards other available objects even the individual's own body. Although this behaviour no longer provides the nutrition and contact that should come from the natural mother-directed behaviour, it continues to provide a state of psychophysiological arousal. Thus digit sucking or self-hugging will occur when an individual is anxious or distressed: the same circumstances in which an animal will return to the mother if reared in this way. Stimulation-seeking behaviours will manifest themselves in a variety of ways depending on the available options afforded by the environment.

Undoubtedly, however, a long-term captive breeding programme will be most effective if it seeks to provide individuals that are raised by their natural mothers in a social group that is approximately the size and demographic composition found for that species in its natural environment. However raising animals in quasi-normal social groups may be impossible in some settings, for example where the wild population is under threat and the numbers in captivity are low. Also there may be individual infants that are weak or have been rejected by their mothers, thus some infants may still not have the experience of being raised in a normal social setting for a valid reason. If this is the case then a social setting must be provided that is as near as possible to the natural condition and is appropriate to the developmental status of the individual. While it may be acceptable to raise an animal alone for health or research reasons, it is not the way to create a self-sustaining, adaptable, captive population.

The type and number of companions will influence social development; the animal's age when these companions are first available, the duration and frequency of access to them and the conditions under which this access is provided. A two-phase management system of mother rearing followed by extensive peer experience offers advantages of being cost effective and practical for breeding colonies of macaques. This system will produce individuals that satisfy the aims of a long-term management programme. When they leave the mother, juveniles should be provided with ample peer experience in compatible social groups of four or more animals. A larger group will provide more stimulation, and explorative behaviour will be encouraged by the provision of certain toys, climbing apparatus and other enclosure devices. Larger groups also reduce the development of excessive infantile clinging and social dependence. Animals should be monitored closely for signs of high levels of aggression, fear, self-clasping, excessive social clinging and other signs of poor adaptation. Positive signs include social and object play and species-typical patterns of sexual behaviour, which in rhesus macaques appear long before puberty. Infant monkeys will form strong attachments not only to other members of the species if separated from their mother, but also to immovable objects such as cloth-covered cylinders used as surrogate mothers. However, apart from providing emotional security, these surrogates do not provide any benefit and the social development of these animals remains impaired; although an interactive surrogate, such as a mechanically driven device, produced animals that exhibited less stereotypies and were more adaptable (Harlow *et al.* 1971).

Many experimental procedures require gaining access to the individual animal but, since primates are intelligent, they can readily be trained to provide researchers with the opportunity to gain access to them even if they are living in social groups. Social inter-action is a significant variable in regulating behaviour and will therefore affect neuro-physiological parameters of primates, which may affect the result of some scientific procedures. However, the neurological model should be based on a normal animal with a defined experimental state of abnormality; any variation introduced by sociality will have less negative effect on the model than the effect of studying a psychologically disturbed animal. The benefits of working on a model based on a more natural condition, within normal parameters, must be balanced against the increase in variability that social living may produce (Reinhardt 2004). Experimantal results from such individuals may not be able to be considered as statistically independent. It may therefore be necessary to increase the number of animals used to account for this, which will increase the overall costs (both financial and ethical) of the experiment, but the overall cost in welfare to the individual will be reduced. It is recognised that the number of animals to be used can sometimes be reduced if additional suffering is allowed to be caused to fewer animals, but in the UK the method licensed will be the one judged to cause the least suffering or distress to the individual (Home Office Guidance on the Animals (Scientific Procedures) Act 1986 para 5.15).

Social subordination may be associated with symptoms of persistent stress such as reproductive inhibition in some species (see Chapter 8); it is not the case that subordination is associated with chronic stress or reproductive dysfunction in all primates. Squirrel monkeys that live without same-sex companions will conceive less often and produce less viable offspring than females that live in social groups including other females. Both dominant and subordinate females benefit reproductively from their association with one another. Similarly, well-being for both dominant and subordinate male squirrel monkeys appears to be enhanced by living with one another.

PRIMATE BEHAVIOUR

All those who work with non-human primates should have training in understanding their behaviour. This will assist in predicting their actions and thus reduce the risk of injury. Basic background information includes the cognitive ability of the species, manual dexterity and leaping ability. On top of this, detailed knowledge of the individual animal's particular idiosyncrasies will assist in the development of a care programme for that animal that is tailored to its needs and does not put the care staff at unnecessary risk.

Species-specific behaviours

Strepsirhines

These are relatively small primates and do not pose a risk of serious physical injury and are generally not aggressive. However, the bite of the slow loris may be of concern since it contains a toxic mix of salivary and glandular secretions (Alterman 1995). Strepsirhines are inquisitive creatures and may leap considerable distances onto people who enter their enclosure for a closer look, so personnel should be prepared for such encounters.

New World monkeys

In general these species are not aggressive and do not respond to direct eye contact in an aggressive way. However they will resist restraint. The callitrichids have sharp claws and incisors and the cebids have sharp canine teeth which can inflict damage. They have good memories and well-developed visual, olfactory and auditory perception, and may form likes and dislikes for individual members of staff. The callitrichids are territorial and threatening behaviour will be shown by an arching of the back, stiff-legged walk, presentation of the testes or chest display, sometimes with piloerection.

Old World monkeys

Many of these species have a combination of well-developed cognitive ability, good body strength for their size and excellent manipulative skills. This can make them expert at escaping from their enclosures. Macaques have very well-developed visual capabilities and visual signals are important in communication, so coloration, facial expression and body posture are used for conspecific communication and mate choice (Waitt *et al.* 2003). The importance of visual stimuli must be recognised by those working with them, if they are not to give incorrect messages to the animals and provoke inappropriate responses that might increase risk. For example, direct eye contact may be perceived as a threat and elicit an aggressive response. Lack of knowledge on the part of personnel working with primates can lead to inadvertent communication of threat by direct eye contact or sudden arm movements. Since they are social animals, a perceived threat by a human to one member of the group may elicit aggression from others in the troupe. Basic training of personnel in primate behaviour will decrease the risk of primate aggressive actions in response to inappropriate human behaviour (see Figure 7.1).

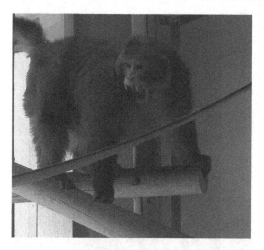

Figure 7.1   Threat response from a rhesus macaque.

MODIFICATION OF BEHAVIOUR

All training techniques for non-human primates should depend principally on positive reinforcement. The proximity of carers is readily established by the positive reinforcement produced by feeding times. Rooms may be cleaned out and feeding done with the animals in the rooms. At such feeding times staff should positively reinforce the development of a social relationship with the animals. Animals will then become relaxed in the presence of the staff, will not show threatening behaviour and females with newly born infants will be relaxed enough to bring them down while foraging on the floor in close proximity to staff (Wolfensohn 2004). Sufficient time should be allocated each day for the staff to spend with the animals (see Figure 7.2).

All staff should be trained in the basics of operant conditioning techniques, they should be capable of implementing simple training protocols and incorporating refinement into their interactions with the animals whenever they carry out husbandry or medical procedures. Training is not something that is just done in a training session, but is a methodology that is incorporated into the daily routine. In a proactive behavioural-management programme the animals are given the opportunity and encouraged to participate voluntarily in certain activities and procedures. The care staff give clear cues for the required response and reinforce those responses when they occur and, to increase the successful outcome, the animals are given plenty of opportunity to carry out that desired behaviour. Staff must plan ahead to prepare animals for veterinary or research procedures. This requires the cooperation and coordination of a number of different groups of staff: veterinary staff, care staff, research staff, and often the input of the ethical review committee and senior managers. Sometimes the opinion of these varied and diverse groups will be at odds and cooperation will not be easy. An overall manager of the programme will have the vital role of team leader and negotiator – diplomatic and personnel skills will be as important as any understanding of the non-human primate

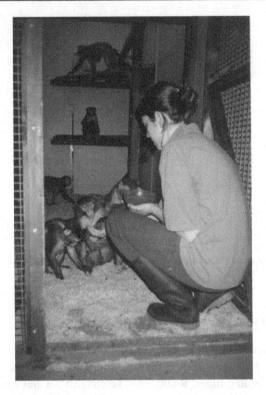

Figure 7.2   Positive interaction with staff.

behaviour. The relationship between the personnel involved in the behavioural-management programme is recognised as being important to its success (Rice *et al*. 2002).

The animal care staff represent the largest part of the behavioural management team since they observe and provide the care for the animal on a daily basis and will be the eyes and ears of the team manager, whether that is a veterinary surgeon or a specialist primatologist. They will work with the environmental enrichment apparatus, setting it up and maintaining it and providing feedback on its effectiveness, use and failings. The team manager must have an open mind to assess real risks and differentiate them from perceived risks; this should be an on-going analysis even after a system has been adopted for use.

Environmental enrichment and positive reinforcement training will assist in addressing the behavioural, psychological, social and physical needs of primates in a captive situation. These need to be combined with sound facility design and operational procedures that can respond to change in a timely manner. In this way, a behavioural management programme as part of an integrated proactive approach to animal welfare will have many benefits for the animals, the staff and, in a research facility, for the science as well.

It is argued that for psychological well-being the same environment should be provided as the animal would experience in natural surroundings. However this would also impose stress, disease, hunger, exposure to the elements and predation, which would not be acceptable in the captive environment. Therefore efforts to improve psychological well-being will utilise such things as comfort, companionship, reaction to challenge and control (choice) (Novak & Suomi 1988). It is not sufficient to attempt to provide a natural environment without thought, since nature is not concerned with psychological well-being, and primates maintained in a captive environment will differ significantly from their wild counterparts. Much better, is something that enriches the research subject and improves the science, if that is the justification for their captivity – examples of these are training and the use of video tasks (Washburn & Rumbaugh 1992).

Early reports of human–monkey interaction note concerns on time required for the human interaction and the potential concomitant increase in staff costs. Human interaction could be enriching for the primate or for macaques it may be threatening and therefore stressful. It is vital to understand primate facial expressions and body language since there are different interpretations of facial signals, e.g. retraction of lips over the teeth (a 'smile' in human terms) is an affiliative signal for chimpanzees and humans, but for macaques this facial signal communicates fear and/or submission (Bayne *et al.* 1993). A direct stare is interpreted as a threat to a macaque, but not a chimpanzee. Therefore any interaction needs to be based on a full understanding of the audio and visual cues specific to that primate species. There is the potential of risk to staff from the interaction, either to health from zoonoses, or the possibility of wounding (see also Chapter 3). Some infections can be transferred bidirectionally and there may therefore be a risk to the animal population. But early studies (Bayne *et al.* 1993) using an A-B-A (baseline – treatment – post-treatment) design showed that something as simple as giving monkeys a food treat either directly off the hand, or in a food box, and spending just 2 minutes per day with each animal resulted in significant modification to behaviours and stereotypic behaviours were consistently reduced. Investing extra time with the monkeys and using their signals for communication (lip smacking, avoiding direct eye contact and submissive body postures) and the provision of certain supplementary foods can result in a significant reduction in undesirable behaviours. The effects of these benefits appeared to be protracted and there was reduction of the pathology even after this enrichment is removed (A-B-A design). Even this minimal type of programme should be implemented since it will have positive benefits, is relatively low cost, and is easy to implement.

Once the close presence of humans is established, the animals' behaviour can be modified. First very simple tasks are achieved, such as getting the monkey to come to a fixed point for feeding, then, for example, running it through a tunnel or into another area for feeding or, in due course, for catching. This should be combined with a verbal command. Most facilities are already carrying out this type of behaviour modification, even if inadvertently. The shout of 'Come on, feed time!' or the clattering sound of the feed trolley will usually bring the animals running to the same point each day, even those that are semi-wild.

Training to permit physical contact

A primate that is used to the presence of people will generally be interested in what is going on and will wish to observe from a safe distance. For most species this will mean getting to a level where it can look down on the proceedings. If the animal is in control of the distance between itself and the person, and can run away if it wants to, it will not feel the need to exhibit threatening behaviour or to defend itself. Before undertaking this training staff must understand primate behaviour and the individual animal, and the study of primate behaviour must be part of the staff development programme (see Chapter 3). For positive reinforcement it is beneficial to use fruit since this is 80% water and therefore will not interfere with the nutritional balance of the diet (see Chapter 4). Juveniles will readily come to take fruit and this will also enable them to establish their own social hierarchy without aggression, as they sort out who comes to the front first, second etc. The shyest monkeys at the back will soon learn from their conspecifics and come down as well.

For adults, the process will inevitably take longer and must be subject to careful and continuous assessment to ensure there are no unnecessary risks to staff. It must be recognised that there may be some individuals that are not temperamentally suitable for close contact with humans, but for the commonly used macaque species this is rare. In the authors' experience, an animal's poor adaptive behaviour is usually the result of an inadequate environment and inappropriate interactions with people earlier in the animal's life. Many such animals, when placed in a well-enriched environment, will become reformed characters; the numbers of those that do not should reduce in the future as a better awareness of the animals' needs in infanthood and the juvenile phase results in improved husbandry, so that such problems do not become established.

Training to facilitate procedures

Once the animals respond well, training can begin to facilitate minor procedures such as blood sampling, and rectal swabbing for routine screening. Traditionally, adult macaques over 3 kg in weight have been restrained by chemical means for minor procedures, such as blood sampling. The administration of sedatives is carried out while the animals are held securely in a crush cage (squeeze back or push front) (see Figure 2.2) or have been captured in a net. A disadvantage of these methods is that the monkey may suffer physical injury particularly to fingers, toes or tail. The potential adverse side effects of the tranquilliser drugs are well documented including hypothermia and alterations in cardiovascular physiology (Flecknell 1996). Undoubtedly such methods cause some degree of stress to the animal and there is scope to refine the methodology to reduce this stress. Training methods using adapted crush cages to encourage the animal to come forward to present a limb for sampling have been described by Reinhardt et al. (2002).

Once a positive response is established, the animals may be trained to stand for intramuscular injections. A method for doing this is as follows. Three staff enter the room, one (A) carrying a catching net, one (B) carrying a syringe and a titbit such as peanut, chocolate drop or piece of dried pasta, the third (C) to act as look out for A and B. Using a three-pronged approach the individual monkey to be trained is singled out from the group. The animal's natural tendency is to move upwards and into the corner of the room and its attention will focus on person A with the net. Person B quietly approaches the animal, showing the syringe and feeds the titbit. The three staff then withdraw. This is repeated daily or twice daily. Once the animal is confident and does not move away, the syringe is shown, then moved to touch the animal's rump and held there for a few seconds before the titbit is given. This is then repeated daily or twice daily. Most animals can be sucessfully trained within less than a week. Reinforcement training is then carried out initially at weekly intervals then at increasing intervals depending on the individual and the clinical/husbandry requirements to make injections (Figure 7.3). Some animals will retain the training without any reinforcement and stand quietly for injections after as many as 6 months.

The method of training employs a subtle combination of positive (the titbit) and negative (the threat of the net) reinforcement. However the net is never used and is simply there to focus the animal's attention. Interestingly animals that have never experienced the use of the net respond to it in the same way as animals that have a history of having previously been netted for capture. The positive reinforcement for this type of procedure is not usually fruit but something more appealing. Only very small quantities are used so that there is no disturbance of the nutritional balance. Once the training is established, use of the net becomes unnecessary. If sedatives, rather than treatments such as antibiotics, are being administered the animal remains under constant observation while the drug takes effect and care is taken to ensure that it does not fall and injure itself.

Juvenile animals that are used to interacting with staff at feeding times may be caught by hand and habituated to sit comfortably on the handler's knee and receive a similar titbit when minor procedures are carried out (see Figure 7.4a, b and c). Juveniles of the larger species may attempt to play nip or orally explore the hands used to apply gentle restraint, so the use of protective gloves made of material such as Kevlar® is beneficial.

Training non-human primates to cooperate during venipuncture in their familiar home environment can eliminate significant stress responses. In many laboratory studies, blood sampling by venipuncture is a routine activity and many animal care managers

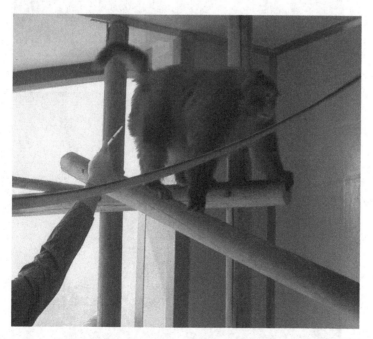

Figure 7.3 Trained rhesus standing for injection.

assume that blood collection requires single-housing and squeezing (and stressing) the primate subjects. Reinhardt (2001) and Reinhardt *et al.* (2002) have demonstrated simple training procedures that are based on positive interaction between the caretaker and primates. Training was based on positive reinforcement with food-treats and vocal praise, consistent firmness, gentleness and patience. The total time investment per male ranged: from 16 to 63 min (mean: 39 min) and from 15 to 45 min (mean: 34 min) for the

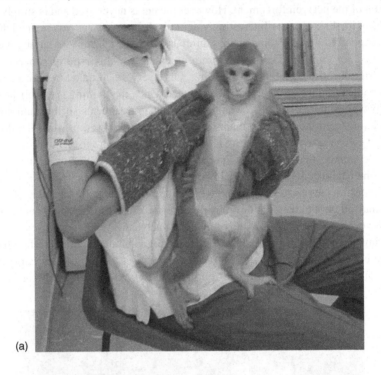

(a)

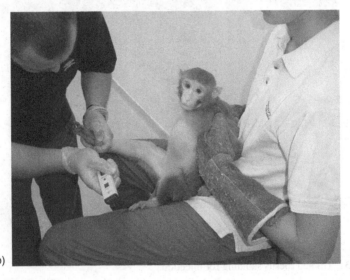

(b)

Figure 7.4   (Continued).

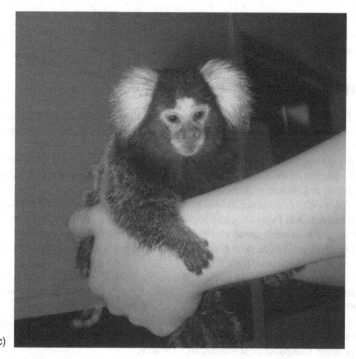

(c)

Figure 7.4 (a) Manual restraint of a rhesus; (b) Restraint for heel prick blood sampling and (c) Handling a marmoset.

stump-tailed females. It took 1–2 min from entering an animal room to the completion of blood collection. The same authors demonstrated how the macaques responded to non-threatening vocal commands and entered a transport cage of their own accord and one at a time. Once trained, each of the males cooperated during blood collection, not only with the trainer but also with the attending care personnel and unfamiliar, yet competent people. If such a trained macaque refuses to take food from the hand of a certain member of staff, their appointment to this type of work should be questioned.

When animals are taken out of their group for a procedure such as blood sampling, reward should not just be given to the individual but to the entire group on its return. Throwing a handful of food such as Rice Krispies or CoCo Pops into the substrate when the individual is put back will compensate the group for the temporary disruption and occupy them so the individual will not be mobbed on its return, smoothing out any possible altercations.

A well-designed behavioural management programme can be a useful tool to reduce risks associated with working with primates. Animals that exhibit behavioural pathology resulting from inadequate captive conditions can be unpredictable and aggressive and will thus present a hazard and high level of risk to workers. It is possible to use drug therapy to reduce the incidence of behavioural pathology (Macy *et al.* 2000), but if animals are maintained in a state of well-being so that they express species-typical behaviour they will be more predictable and worker safety will improve. If the animals also associate the presence of such workers with positive experiences like food treats or cognitive activities, they will be affiliative rather then aggressive towards the staff and will learn to cooperate in the activity. Care must be taken that the animals do not form social hierarchies that inadvertently involve the staff through acts of aggression or submission.

FURTHER READING

Alterman, L. (1995) Toxins and toothcombs: potential allospecific chemical defense in *Nycticebus* and *Perodicticus*. In: *Creatures of the Dark* (eds L. Alterman, G. Doyle & M.K. Izand) pp. 413–424. Plenum Press, New York.

Bayne K.A.L., Dexter S.L., & Strange G.M. (1993) The effects of food treat provisioning and human interaction on the behavioural well-being of rhesus monkeys (*Macaca mulatta*). *Contemporary Topics in Laboratory Animal Science*, **32**, 6–9.

Flecknell, P.A. (1996) *Laboratory Animal Anaesthesia*, 2nd edn. Academic Press, London.

IPS (1993) International Primatological Society: International guidelines for the acquisition, care and breeding of nonhuman primates. *Primate Report* (special issue).

Harlow, H.F., Harlow, M.K. & Suomi, S.J. (1971) From thought to therapy: Lessons from a primate laboratory. *American Scientist*, **59**, 538–549.

Luttrell, L., Acker, L., Urben, M., & Reinhardt, V. (1994) Training a large troop of rhesus macaques to cooperate during catching: Analysis of the time investment. *Animal Welfare*, **3**, 135–140. http://www.awionline.org/Lab_animals/biblio/aw5train.htm

Macy, J.D., Beattie, T.A., Morgenstern, S.E. & Arnsten, A.F.T. (2000) Use of guanfacine to control self-injurious behaviour in two rhesus macaques (*Macaca mulatta*) and one baboon (*Papio anubis*). *Comparative Medicine*, **50**, 419–425.

Novak, M.A. & Suomi S.J. (1988) Psychological well-being of primates in captivity. *American Journal of Psychology*, **43**, 765–773.

NRC (1997) *The Psychological Well-being of Non-human Primates*. National Research Council. National Academy Press, Washington D.C.

Prestcott, M. & Buchanan-Smith, H. (2003) Training non-human primates using positive reinforcement techniques. *Journal of Applied Animal Welfare Science*, **6**, 157–261.

Reinhardt, V. (2001) Training pair-housed rhesus males to cooperate during blood collection. Primate Enrichment Network (PEN); http://primate-enrichment.net Item No. A107.

Reinhardt, V. (2004) Common husbandry-related variables in biomedical research with animals. *Laboratory Animals*, **38**, 213–235.

Reinhardt, V., Buchanan-Smith, H.M., & Prescott, M.J. (2002) Training macaques to voluntarily co-operate during two common procedures: Blood collection and capture of group-housed animals. In: *XIXth Congress of the International Primatological Society, Abstracts – Caring for Primates*, pp. 182–183, Abstract. Mammalogical Society of China, Beijing, China.

Rice, T.R., Walden, S., Laule, G.E., & Heidbrink, G.A. (2002) Behavioural management: it's everyone's job. *Contemporary Topics in Laboratory Animal Science*, **41**, 58–61.

Waitt, C., Little, A., Wolfensohn, S., *et al.* (2003) Evidence from rhesus macaques suggests that male colouration plays a role in female mate choice. *Proceedings of the Royal Society of London B*, **270** (S2), 144–146.

Washburn, D.A. & Rumbaugh, D.M. (1992) Investigations of rhesus monkey video-task performance: evidence for enrichment. *Contemporary Topics in Laboratory Animal Science*, **31**, 6–10.

Wolfensohn, S. (2004) *Social Housing of Large Primates: Methodology for refinement of husbandry and management*. ATLA 32, Supplement 1, 149–151.

Chapter 8
Breeding

A number of texts give extensive coverage the parameters of primate reproduction, such as the duration of events, adult and neonate weights, growth curves, infant feeding, weaning and physical and behavioural development (e.g. Kirkwood & Stathatos 1992; Poole 1999). This chapter will avoid duplicating this effort and instead concentrate on general themes and advice relating to primate reproduction and breeding. It is important to understand some of the factors and patterns that influence species-specific life history and reproductive parameters; therefore this chapter will begin by giving a brief overview of patterns of primate social grouping and factors that influence reproductive success.

GROUP SYSTEMS AND SIZES

It is important when discussing grouping systems in primates to distinguish between *grouping* or *social* systems and *breeding* or *mating* systems. The highest level of classification is simply whether a species is gregarious (forming groups), such as most haplorhine primates, or non-gregarious like most of the strepsirhine species plus a few notable haplorhines including the orang-utan (*Pongo pygmaeus*). It is a mistake, however, to confuse gregarious/non-gregarious social systems with social/asocial behaviour. Non-gregarious species still exhibit high levels of social behaviour communicating with and often meeting conspecifics which, for reasons of resource distribution, are forced to lead lives within a social system that is spatially dispersed. Most primate species that are maintained in captivity have gregarious social systems, although the typical size of groups in which they would live in the wild and the mating system exhibited may vary.

It is incorrect to view primate groups simply as a convenient aggregation of individuals for breeding purposes. As Dixson (1998) points out: seasonal breeders (e.g. many New World primates) still form groups year-round, therefore a species' social system is not simply a product of its mating system. However, a mating system can be defined as: 'the general mode of co-ordination, access and interaction between males and females within a specific social grouping; they are embedded in the social system, but are not themselves a definition of sociality' (Lee 1994).

What determines the form of mating system?

Richard Wrangham's (1980) ecological model of female-bonded groups gives perhaps the most broadly accepted explanation of the influence of ecological variables on the patterns of grouping observed in primates, particularly Old World species. Where patches of resources are large enough to be exploited by more than one individual, cooperation and long-term bonding are encouraged to enable effective use of these resources and their protection from extra-group individuals. Primates are highly social animals and typically form groups in which the individuals of one or other sex (usually the females) may be related. However there are both costs and benefits accrued from living in a group (van Schaik 1983; Krebs & Davies 1993; Lee 1994; Strier 2000) and a way of reducing the impact of the costs associated with group living is to live with close relatives. Thereby any cost accrued by losing out to a fellow group member (e.g. in feeding or mating resources) or as a product of living in a group (parasites, predation) is in the cause of assisting the survival and success of an individual, through kin selection, with whom genes are shared and so helping to maximise their inclusive fitness (Krebs & Davies 1993). These can therefore be described as kin-bonded groups and in primates these are typically female kin-bonded groups monopolising feeding resources – the major constraint on female reproductive potential (the ability to attain reproductive condition, gestate and feed offspring). Wrangham, in his model, points out that the distribution of males is then superimposed onto that of the females as access to females is the major limiter on male reproductive potential. The distribution of males around these groups of females is affected by other factors such as male–male competition and predation risk (van Schaik & Hostermann 1994). The variation observed in grouping patterns between species and indeed between populations of the same species is due to differences in the quality and density of resources, as well as other factors such as disease and predation threat as well as environmental stress (e.g. thermoregulation). An excellent treatment of the variation in primate societies and the different strategies adopted by different species in balancing the costs and benefits of group living with attempts to maximise individual reproductive success and inclusive fitness can be seen in the contributions of several authors in Smuts *et al.* (1987).

Clearly, the nature of relatedness within groups determines the general pattern of emigration and dispersal. For example if groups are made up of related females then this means that to avoid inbreeding, maturing males must disperse while females remain resident in related lineages or matrilines, e.g. in the baboons (*Papio* spp.) and macaques (*Macaca* spp.). In these groups of related females higher levels of cooperative behaviour are seen among the females than among the males. In the rare instances (e.g. the chimpanzee, *Pan troglodytes*) where females disperse from their natal group, patrilines of related males remain resident and the pattern of cooperation within the group is largely between males.

Classification of primate mating systems

Primate mating systems can be classified into the following four broad categories:

- *Monogamy*: One male and one female mate for the length of a reproductive event and thereby ensure paternity (e.g. titi monkeys, *Callicebus* spp.; gibbons, *Hylobates* spp.).
- *Polyandry*: Several males mate with one female for the length of a reproductive event (e.g. saddle-back tamarin, *Saguinus fuscicollis*). In those species where polyandry has been recorded, monogamy also exists and may be the primary mating system (Dixson 1998).

- *Single-male harem*: One male mates with a number of females, which are kin-bonded. Males attempt paternity certainty by excluding other males and in some instances through infanticide of infants under a certain age.
- *Multimale unit*: Matings may be promiscuous (several males with several females) or monopolised (one male with several females) through dominance. Groups may be either male-bonded (e.g. chimpanzee, *Pan troglodytes*) or female-bonded (e.g. macaques, *Macaca* sp.).

Levels of grouping in addition to those described here do exist and are of two main types. First, and more likely in species where groups are male-bonded (e.g. chimpanzee, *Pan troglodytes*; and spider monkeys, *Ateles* sp.) communities are formed in a communally defended, geographically distinct area. For foraging, the community divides into smaller parties of variable size and composition. These are known as fission–fusion societies. Second, in some species (e.g. the gelada, *Theropithecus gelada*; and hamadryas baboon, *Papio hamadryas*) a number of stable, social, breeding units may come together into larger groups, known as bands or herds, for social or sleeping purposes. There are also instances in which individuals of either sex, across a range of mating systems have been recorded soliciting and achieving matings with non-dominant and even non-group members (Strier 2000).

In systems other than where monogamy exists, males must compete actively for access to females and it is their degree and duration of success at doing this that plays a major role in their reproductive success (see Strier 2000, for a full review of male reproductive strategies). In single-male systems each male aims to achieve monopoly over a group of breeding females. Generally this requires the displacement of the existing harem male, typically entailing violence. Alternatively, he can join the group as a non-breeding, subordinate male with the hope of acquiring sole mating rights at a later date (e.g. hamadryas baboon, *Papio hamadryas*). In the gelada (*Theropithecus gelada*) these 'followers' will form relationships with females within the group and may then lead these females away to form a new group (Stammbach 1987).

In multimale systems the competition for females takes place when they become reproductively receptive. This competition is primarily though dominance status derived from contests. However, the relationship between male dominance and reproductive success in primates is not a clear-cut one (de Ruiter & van Hoof 1993), as the proportion of matings monopolised by the dominant male may not be reflected in the paternity of the offspring, determined from DNA fingerprinting (Dixson 1998). This can be affected by female mate choice, the timing (during the ovarian cycle) of the mating as well as post-mating effects such as the presence and success of any mate guarding, sperm competition and copulatory plugs (Dixson 1998). While a number of studies have not found strong correlation between male dominance rank and reproductive success in primates, de Ruiter and van Hoof (1993) do report a strong relationship in their study of wild long-tailed macaques (*Macaca fascicularis*). They point out that such studies of wild populations do report a positive correlation, whereas many of the studies where a positive relationship, if any, is not demonstrable are conducted in captivity – where this may be due to particular constraints of captivity (reduced space and prevention of natural migration patterns) and group size.

A male's lifetime reproductive success will be determined by his ability to maximise his rank early in his reproductive life as well as by the duration of his reproductive lifespan.

Some males, however, opt for alternative strategies and (e.g. in baboons) form special affiliative bonds with females in the group, often fostered by assisting with infant care duties, which may afford the male future mating access. Also if a male's rank is insufficient to enable him to gain access to females in competition against a higher ranking male then he may form one, or more, alliances with other males in order to out-compete the dominant male. This may subsequently entail the sharing of the spoils between the alliance members. The strategy of alliance formation may also be employed by a male just coming off his prime to extend the duration of his dominance.

When examining potential or realised reproductive success in primates as with other mammals, it is important to consider four key elements (Clutton-Brock 1988):

- survival to reproductive age
- duration of reproductive lifespan
- productivity during reproductive lifespan
- survival of offspring to reproductive age.

First, the individual must be able to survive to breeding age and this is dependent on the health and condition of the mother, the growth rate of the infant and factors such as predation, disease and accidental death. Second, the duration of the reproductive lifespan is, in turn, determined by the age at which the animal first reproduces and the age at which it ceases to be able to reproduce due to mortality or age-specific effects. Internal physiological effects may also determine the end of the reproductive life (e.g. the onset of menopause in humans). Third, productivity over the reproductive lifespan is determined by effects on fertility: environmental (e.g. food abundance and quality), social (e.g. male loss of status and displacement from a harem by a younger, stronger male), lactational (e.g. duration and cost of lactation to the mother, affecting the timing of her return to reproductive condition – a complex interaction discussed later in this chapter) and genetic (e.g. natural variation in fertility between individuals). Finally, to ensure their genetic contribution to succeeding generations any offspring produced must, themselves, be able to survive to reproduce. This is constrained by their own ability to grow and develop and is therefore also a factor of the condition of their mother as well as their ability to avoid mortality from predation, disease etc.

It is also the case that in mammals the variation in reproductive success among males can be much greater than that in females. In primates, at any one reproductive event females produce only one offspring (though this may be twins, triplets or even quadruplets in callitrichids) regardless of how many males she mates with, whereas over this same period of time a male could possibly father hundreds of offspring. This variance in male reproductive success has implications for sexual selection, mating strategies and patterns of parental investment (Bateman's Principle: Bateman 1948).

PRIMATE FERTILITY

A natural variation exists in fertility, both at the interpopulation as well as the intrapopulation level, as a result of differences in internal factors such as the genetics, energetics and stress, as well as externally determined factors such as nutrition and disease.

Nutritional influences

In primates that are seasonal breeders or where food availability varies there can be a marked effect on fertility in females. In environments where more energy is available (better resources) the age at first reproduction is earlier, conception is more probable (higher birth rate), inter-birth intervals are shorter and there are better infant survival rates (Dunbar 1987; Lee 1987). In poor quality environments populations may undergo a change in the sex ratio, which may have the knock-on effect of a reduction in population growth rate (Lee 1988).

Environmental influences

Females need to maintain at least a minimum body weight (or levels of body fat) in order to either begin (at puberty) or resume (e.g. after a reproductive event) ovulatory cycling. Their ability to do this may be affected by environmental stress or poor immunological function. Environmental stress, in the form of raised energy costs in food and/or water searches compounded by carrying infants and lactating, also contributes directly to the challenges facing a female in achieving the required condition for fertility. There may also be social constraints imposed through hierarchical dominance that not only induce stress but also limit the amount of food a female may take (Harcourt 1987). Finally she may have extra costs resulting from the sex of the infant she produces, as in many primate species (e.g. baboons and macaques) there is a substantial sexual dimorphism in body size and there are therefore higher costs in providing for the continued growth of male offspring.

The distribution of the quality of resources in the environment may be subject to a marked seasonality. In tropical forests this may be a wet/dry season difference, and in more temperate regions or at higher altitudes the pattern may be one that follows spring/summer/autumn/winter, either way this may have a marked effect on the availability and quality of important food resources. In response to this some species, or populations of species, have become seasonal breeders; only breeding at times of year that ensure the infants are born at a time of abundant, high quality resources. This reduces the impact of lactation on the condition of the female, allowing her to become fertile again sooner, as well as providing good conditions for the early growth of the infant. The rhesus (*Macaca mulatta*) is a seasonal breeder, where reproduction appears to be triggered by changes in day length (Baskerville 1999). The importance of day length is supported by an interesting observation in a captive rhesus population in Brazil, outside the natural range of this species which in its natural state lives exclusively in the northern hemisphere. In the Brazilian colony there is an inversion of the breeding season, with births occurring when the days are longer between October and April compared with March to September in the northern hemisphere (Gomes & Bicca-Marques 2003). Provided that resources are of sufficient quality for a female to attain the necessary condition for fertility, the major recurring influence on female fertility is lactation. This acts in three ways: through the inhibition of ovulation, the draining effect on maternal condition, and as a source of energy for the infant's growth (and is initially the only source) (Lee 1987).

Social influences

There are often strong social influences on an animal's fertility, particularly in those primate species that live in groups. One of the ways that primates moderate the potentially very injurious process of competing for resources, such as food, nest sites or mates, is through the development of dominance hierarchies. Dominance rank is attained and maintained through often highly stylised displays of strength, or in the case of some macaque species (e.g. Japanese and rhesus macaques; *Macaca fuscata* and *M. mulatta*) through the inheritance of maternal rank. Thereby the amount of fully aggressive competition for limited resources is greatly reduced or even removed, as is therefore the potential for the damaging of relationships that have taken considerable investment to establish (de Waal 1989). There is evidence that females with higher dominance rank breed earlier and produce more offspring per year (Harcourt 1987). Competition for limited resources can also result in cooperative infant rearing, with often unrelated, non-breeding individuals contributing to the rearing of infants in exchange for future access to resources, for example the carrying of infants by helpers in the callitrichids (Dunbar 1995).

Where access to mates is the subject of competition this can often lead to strong sexual dimorphism particularly in body size where contests within a sex (usually males) determines status and therefore access to mates. The action of strong selective pressures for large, powerful males can be clearly seen in a number of primate species (e.g. mandrill, *Mandrillus sphinx* (Setchell *et al.* 2001) and orang-utan, *Pongo pygmaeus*) (Dixson 1998). The more powerful the male, the higher his social status and thereby the greater his access to mates. His power may also enable him totally to exclude other males from the group to monopolise matings, but females may also manipulate group composition by rejecting or accepting males and by tolerating one or more males in the group. In some cases hormonal suppression of fertility, as seen in the callitrichids, functions to decrease competition for mates within a social group.

NATURAL SUPPRESSION OF FERTILITY

As described above, a number of primate species use social dominance and status to improve their reproductive success, primarily through behavioural (e.g. aggression and harassment) and/or physiological (e.g. pheromones and endocrine pathways) means. In some animals a reproductive monopoly may be maintained through the infanticide of other individuals' offspring (Abbott 1988).

Reproductive suppression of subordinates (both male and female) is a key feature of reproduction and breeding in the smallest of the New World primates; the marmosets (*Callithrix* spp.) and tamarins (*Saguinus* spp.) (Abbott 1988). In groups of these primates only a few of the adults reproduce, and contraception, through conflict within the group, is achieved in the subordinate animals. The dominant male and dominant female maintain a tight pair-bond monopolising reproduction within the group. Typically twins are produced, but litters of up to four are known in captivity. Parenting support, largely in the form of infant carrying, is received from the non-breeding subordinates within the group (Dunbar 1995). Infertility is imposed on other group members through both behavioural (social aggression) and physiological (pheromonal) mechanisms (Abbott 1988).

Reproductive suppression of females

A valuable review of the factors controlling reproductive suppression in subordinate female common marmosets (*Callithrix jacchus*) was published by Abbott *et al*. (1998). The authors describe how some aspects of reproductive suppression may be achieved through physiological mechanisms and this can clearly be seen in the insufficient production of gonadotrophin, producing an anovulatory state in subordinate animals (see Figure 8.1). By removing a subordinate from the presence of a dominant animal an increase in the production of luteinising hormone (LH) (within 1–4 days) by the pituitary gland can be affected, accompanied by restarting the ovulatory cycle (see Figure 8.2). This decrease in LH does not appear to be caused by suppression of the secretion of GnRH (gonadotrophin-releasing hormone) by the hypothalamus as levels are similar in subordinate and dominant females. Abbott *et al*. (1998) also state that 'Factors such as reduced pituitary gonadotrophin responsiveness to GnRH, insufficient priming of pituitary gonadotrophins, or a combination of factors leading to reduced pituitary sensitivity to GnRH may be responsible for the hypogonadotrophic condition of subordinates.' The low levels of LH in subordinates are not related to blood cortisol or prolactin levels nor

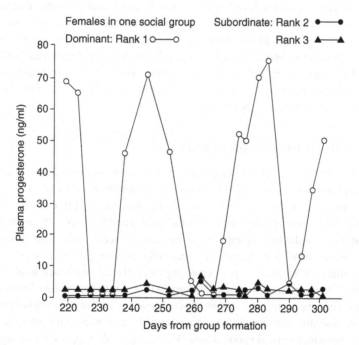

Figure 8.1 An example of plasma progesterone levels in a dominant common marmoset female and her two subordinates. The period of time shown starts at the end of a luteal phase for the dominant female and continues through her next three ovarian cycles, finishing in the mid-luteal phase of the third cycle. Reprinted with permission from Abbott (1989).

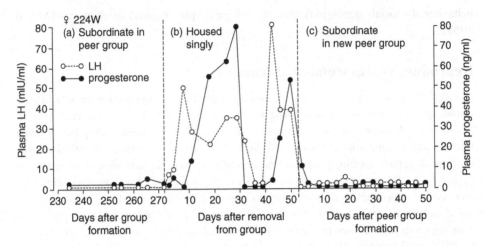

Figure 8.2   Changes in the plasma levels of progesterone and luteinizing hormone (LH) in a female common marmoset (*Callithrix jacchus*) over three phases: (a) as a subordinate in a peer group; (b) singly housed; (c) as a subordinate in a new peer group. Reprinted with permission from Abbott (1988).

to weight loss features that would indicate stress. This drop in circulating LH is reversed when subordinates are reintroduced to the dominant female and it appears that the primary cues for this suppression in subordinates appear to be olfactory ones, from the dominant female. Abbott (1989) found that there were increases in both plasma progesterone and LH when female common marmosets (*Callithrix jacchus*) were removed from either an established peer group, in which they were subordinate, to single housing, or when removed from their mothers; an effect that was reversed on the return of the animal to its original social environment (Abbott 1989).

Reproductive suppression of males

Baker *et al.* (1999) have demonstrated in common marmosets (*Callithrix jacchus*) that while the reproductive activity of subordinate males within their social group is substantially less than that of the dominant male, this is not due to differences in cortisol or testosterone levels, as these are the same in the fathers and their sons. Their work demonstrates that the reproductive suppression is instead an incest-avoidance strategy as sons performed sexual behaviour equally as frequently as their fathers in tests with novel, unrelated females; whereas they performed significantly less with their mothers than did their father. When presented with a novel female together the response of both father and son was reduced, suggesting an element of male–male competition. In wild or free-ranging populations subordinate males have been observed to mate with extra-group females and are known to produce normal spermatozoa. Therefore, while suppression of reproduction of subordinate male callitrichids within groups may not be due to dominance suppression, it can rather be seen as avoidance of mating with familiar females coupled with a degree of father–son competition (Baker *et al.* 1999). The role of female primates in aggressively rejecting mating attempts is also a way of restricting reproduction in subordinate males.

REPRODUCTIVE CYCLES

Female primates, from the onset of puberty, experience cyclical fluctuations in hormones due to the maternal factors of pregnancy and lactation, as well as the usual ovarian cycle and these changes may be reflected in both behaviour and appearance (e.g. sexual swellings). Fraser and Lunn (1999) present a detailed description of the physiological features of reproduction in female non-human primates and their use as models for the study of human reproduction. Figures for primate ovarian cycle length are given in Hendrickx and Dukelow (1995a). Dixson (1998) describes in detail the differences between primate taxa in their reproductive anatomy, both internal and external. Evidence is presented for the role of differences in male and female genital morphology in a species' mate recognition (interspecific) and in sexual selection (intraspecific). While New World and Old World primates share many features, there are nevertheless considerable differences, for example in ovarian size and structure with accompanying effects on reproductive hormones as well as the incidence of menstruation, which is the norm among female Old World monkeys and apes but is rare among New World species (exceptions being the capuchins, *Cebus* spp. and spider monkeys *Ateles* spp.) (Dixson 1998; Hendrickx & Dukelow 1995a). Much is known, through very detailed research, about the menstrual cycle of the rhesus macaque (*Macaca mulatta*) (see Dixson 1998).

There is an absence of externals signals of the occurrence of ovulation in New World species as there is no sexual skin; however in a few species (e.g. squirrel monkeys, *Saimiri* spp.) there is some swelling of the external female genitalia. Some squirrel monkey males also come into a breeding condition in which they are known as 'fatted', putting on substantial amounts of weight on their upper body and further evidence suggests a female mating preference for such males (Mendoza *et al.* 1978).

The size and colour (generally pink) of the sexual skin region in Old World primates may not only indicate the occurrence of ovulation but may also be associated with attractiveness in the context of mate choice, both of females to males and *vice versa* (e.g. in rhesus macaques; Waitt *et al.* 2003). In females the anogenital region is frequently the primary site of sexual skin, but other areas, such as the side of the thighs (e.g. rhesus macaques, *Macaca mulatta*) or the chest (gelada, *Theropithecus gelada*) may be involved. The presence of sexual skin in male primates should also not be overlooked; these areas are often very dramatic and brightly coloured (e.g. the blue of the scrotum of the vervet monkey (*Cercopithecus aethiops*) or the bright red and blue of the nasal skin of the mandrill (*Mandrillus sphinx*)) (Dixson 1998).

In addition to visual signals of reproductive state, communication via auditory and olfactory media is extremely important in many primate species. Dixson (1998) reviews the role of olfactory cues in female sexual attractiveness and these are of greatest importance among primates in the strepsirhines and the New World monkeys. Exceptionally valuable research into the communication of reproductive condition in female primate vocalisations has been conducted by Stuart Semple and colleagues (Semple & McComb 2000). They were able to demonstrate, experimentally, in female Barbary macaques

(*Macaca sylvanus*) that variation in key temporal and frequency parameters of vocalisations varied with reproductive condition and that these changes were perceivable and used by males in attempts to maximise their reproductive success.

The reproductive behaviour of male and female primates may vary considerably across the ovarian cycle, for example in the frequency of ejaculatory mounts in males and the proceptiveness and receptiveness of females. Evidence suggests that changes in the proceptivity behaviour of females, in initiating copulations, may serve as a useful predictor of the day of conception in some species (e.g. rhesus macaque, *Macaca mulatta*; Zehr *et al.* 2000), which may be very valuable for studies where accurate aging of embryos is required.

ARTIFICIAL CONTROL OF REPRODUCTION

Contraception

In some cases it may not be desirable to have primates breeding, and contraceptive strategies may be employed in a number of circumstances:

- genetic management of captive populations, without the need for social disruption caused by the removal of individuals, or the loss of future potentially valuable genetic resources through culling;
- humane control of free-ranging primates in a human–wildlife conflict situation;
- preventing increases in numbers of individuals of non-threatened species, which are not part of captive breeding programmes (e.g. in zoos or wildlife sanctuaries).

Permanent measures may be taken through surgical means, but in most cases a reversible solution is required. Callitrichids, the marmosets and tamarins, are a particular target for contraception in captivity due to the small social groups in which they should be kept (generally a mature pair plus one or two generations of offspring), and their high reproductive output through the production of twins, triplets and occasionally quadruplets. A review of humane control issues and techniques for captive callitrichids is to be found in Sainsbury (1997). The preferred technique is through the use of progestagen implants (0.3–0.5 mg, 10×5 mm, containing 10 mg melengestrol acetate, or with levonorgestrel) or injection (medroxyprogesterone acetate) (Sainsbury 1997). Medroxyprogesterone acetate (DMPA) can be obtained on prescription as Depo-Provera® (Pharmacia) in pre-filled 150 mg/ml 1-ml syringes (dose: – marmosets: 3 mg/kg; macaques: 4–7 mg/kg). To dose marmosets it is best to make a 1:10 dilution by adding 0.1 ml of DMPA to 0.9 ml of water for injection, and then to give 0.1 ml of this dilution per 500 g body weight by deep intramuscular injection. It should be started within 5 days of parturition or any time in non-pregnant females, and is then repeated every 12 weeks. There is no need to separate the female from males or offspring, and the only observed side effect may be mild weight gain.

However there are complications associated with the use of contraceptives. Implants may be lost (as many as 16%), for example by their removal by the recipient. A new implant might not be administered before the end of the effectiveness of an old one, possibly resulting in pregnancy. Implanting an animal may require its separation from group mates for a period, which may have social implications (Sainsbury 1997). More serious implications such as permanent sterility (Sainsbury 1997) and a predisposition with the use of progesterone implants, in macaques, to SIV infection by sexual transmission possibly due to a thinning of the vaginal epithelium (Marx *et al.* 1996) must also be considered.

Further, emergency contraception can be used and has been demonstrated as successful in some primates (especially the rhesus macaque, *Macaca mulatta*) in preventing implantation (Sengupta *et al.* 2003). Additional, valuable information on contraception can be found in the AZA Contraception Advisory Group Recommendations (2003).

Artificial insemination

Artificial insemination is a breeding management strategy that is generally unnecessary in the normal captive breeding of primates. There are two instances where artificial insemination may be required: either as part of a captive breeding programme for an endangered species for genetic management and/or where there may be problems with mating behaviour, or as part of a specific scientific procedure, e.g. involving the use modified sperm.

Artificial insemination has been demonstrated in a range of Old World primate species (Gould & Martin 1986), including in the rhesus macaque (Dede & Plentl 1966). Despite the absence, in many New World primate species, of clear external signs of oestrus and ovulation successful artificial insemination has been demonstrated in the common marmoset (*Callithrix jacchus*) using fresh (Morrell *et al.* 1997) or cryopreserved sperm (Morrell *et al.* 1998) for use as a tool in captive breeding programmes. In extreme instances *in vitro* fertilisation (IVF) and embryo transfer may be employed for a number of experimental reasons (Dukelow & Clemens 1999), as well as for genetic management or conservation purposes, for example as in the case of the western lowland gorilla (Pope *et al.* 1997).

PREGNANCY DIAGNOSIS

The diagnosis of pregnancy in primates can be remarkably accurate when carried out by an experienced researcher, technician or veterinary surgeon. Methods include manual palpation (detectable from 16 days in macaques and 30 days in the common marmoset, *Callithrix jacchus*), use of ultrasound imaging (detectable at 16–18 days in the rhesus macaque) (Figures 8.3 and 8.4) and the detection of the hormonal changes that accompany pregnancy and which can be detected in the urine and blood serum (Kirkwood & Stathatos 1992; Hendrickx & Dukelow 1995b). It is also possible to use morphological and endocrine diagnosis to determine the early loss of pregnancy (Hendrickx *et al.* 1999).

PARTURITION

Parturition takes place following a gestation period (e.g. approximately 166 days in the rhesus macaque (*Macaca mulatta*) and yellow baboon (*Papio cynocephalus*), and 144 days in the common marmoset, *Callithrix jacchus*) (Kirkwood & Stathatos 1992).

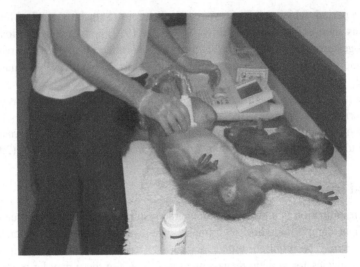

Figure 8.3 Performing an ultrasound examination on a sedated rhesus macaque.

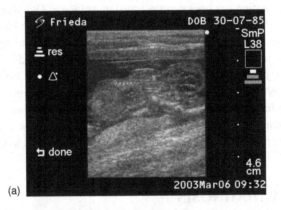

(a)

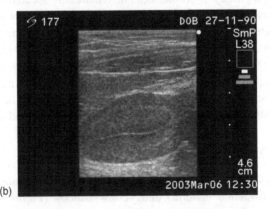

(b)

Figure 8.4 (a) An ultrasound scan, pregnant and (b) an ultrasound scan, non-pregnant.

Hendrickx and Dukelow (1995a) detail many of the hormonal changes that occur during pregnancy and then at parturition. In most primates parturition takes place at night or in the early morning and may last for a variable time depending on the experience of the mother and whether there are any complications. In the rhesus any delivery that takes in excess of 3 hours requires careful monitoring and may require veterinary intervention (Kirkwood & Stathatos 1992).

It is usual for the smaller New World primates to produce multiple births, but this is much rarer in Old World primates (0.06% to 0.5% of births in macaques: Canfield *et al.* 2000), though twins are known to occur (e.g. in the stump-tailed macaque, *Macaca arctoides*; Schrier & Povar 1984). Complications such as the production of conjoined twins are even rarer, but reports do exist, including in the rhesus macaque (Canfield *et al.* 2000).

LACTATION AND WEANING

The production of milk and suckling behaviour is a vital part of the reproductive cycle of primates. It performs several important functions: in the nourishment and providing early immune protection (through colostrum) of the infant; establishing and maintaining the mother–infant bond; and, except in a few species (e.g. marmosets), producing lactational amenorrhea – a period after the birth during which the ovarian cycle is impeded and the mother is prevented from becoming pregnant. While some strepsirhine species have two pairs of mammary glands, monkeys and apes have just one pair from which the newborn infant begins to suckle instinctively within minutes, or just a few hours, after birth (Hendrickx & Dukelow 1995a). Data on the length of the lactation period, as well as nutrition information about the contents of primate milk, for many species are presented in Chapter 4 and in Hendrickx and Dukelow (1995a).

In some instances it may be necessary to consider hand-rearing of an infant, for example if it is rejected by its mother or owing to the death of the mother. The issue of and techniques involved in hand-rearing are discussed in Chapter 4.

In any discussion of weaning, particularly in captive primates, it is necessary to define clearly what is meant by the term weaning. Lactation in the macaque female has all but drawn to an end by 10–11 months, so that the infants would be fully weaned before the birth of the next baby, and at this stage they do not depend on their mother for nutrition. Confusion arises because of the use of the term 'weaning' to describe the cessation of suckling by the mother in unmanaged populations, forming part of her life-history strategy and energy investment pattern; as well as to describe the forcible removal of offspring in captive populations as part of a breeding management or supply strategy. Lee (1999) demonstrates, through comparative studies, that the conflicting requirements of the mother (accelerate weaning) and offspring (prolong suckling) result in the mother terminating suckling at a point determined by the metabolic independence of the offspring, this being a factor of the offspring's body weight at birth and at weaning – the 'metabolic weaning weight'. In rhesus macaques the threshold weaning weight is 1.335 kg (a range of 1.0–1.6 kg), which reflects a constant multiple, 3.4, of the neonate's birth weight (Lee 1999). The same author also notes the constant proportion (within a species) of maternal weight to neonate weight and the presence of a decrease in this proportion in progressively larger primate species. Many of the theoretical issues surrounding weaning strategies and the energetic challenges facing the mother and infant that result in weaning conflict are discussed elsewhere (e.g. Altmann 1980; Lee 1987).

Weaning is not an abrupt event but a process lasting several months. Most infants can feed themselves at 6 months but remain socially dependent on their mothers and return to them when disturbed and to sleep. This period of suckling and gradual weaning is an important time in the development of the infant. It is during this time and shortly after that they begin to learn from their mother and refine the food selection, acquisition and processing skills that will be vital in enabling their feeding independence after weaning (Altmann 1980; Janson & van Schaik 2002). After the first year, juvenile animals can become more and more involved in peer groups, especially the males. Stimulus deprivation in infancy has been shown to have a dramatic impact on the development of young macaques, making them less active, more withdrawn, involved in more clutching and stereotypic behaviour (Harlow *et al.* 1965) as well as having higher basal cortisol levels and showing more fear-disturbance-emotional behaviour than non-deprived control animals (Sacket *et al.* 1973). The National Research Council (NRC, 1997) points out that although the importance of social stimulation during infancy is well established, considerably less is known about the influence of social contact during juvenile and adolescent stages of development. It is therefore important to monitor each animal and if the assessments indicate an incidence of behavioural problems then management regimes, such as weaning age, should be reviewed. It is the continual assessment of behaviour and welfare that is more important that sticking to rigid temporal criteria. For example, if animals are weaned in batches, it is more important to keep a younger animal of, say, 9 months, with its older half siblings of, say, 12 months, with which it has already formed social relationships, than to postpone weaning and introduce it 3 months later to an unknown group. Of course if that individual was for some reason poorly grown then weaning should be delayed. Each animal has to be considered individually.

Since many managers have tried to use temporal criteria for weaning, contradictory opinions abound. The UK Home Office Code of Practice for the housing and care of animals bred for experimental purposes states for macaques 'Young animals must not be weaned at less than six months and 1 kg in body weight, unless on veterinary advice e.g. mother is unable to rear baby. It is preferable not to wean before 12 months of age.' The Universities Federation for Animal Welfare (Poole 1999) states: 'The best compromise is probably to wean most infants at around 6 months, but to leave individuals who are not doing very well with their mothers for a longer period.' However, the International Primatological Society guidelines (IPS 1993) state that 'The young monkey should not normally be separated from its mother at an early age (i.e. at 3–6 months) but should remain in contact for one year to 18 months.' Goo and Fugate (1984) found there were no significant differences in survival to 2 years among groups of rhesus macaques weaned at 6, 8, 10 and 12 months of age. However the authors do report pregnancy rates that are substantially lower than those reported for rhesus in the wild. Reinhardt (2002) points out the absence from the study of a control group that were allowed to remain with their mother beyond the biological weaning age and that the difference between the pregnancy rates reported in these groups compared with the wild is an indication that the loss of the infant has an 'intrinsic impact on the mother's reproductive system'. Reinhardt (2002) also cites a further study in the case against forced weaning: Wallis and Valentine (2001) who found that baboon (*Papio* sp.) mothers whose infants had been forcibly removed (at 6–10 months) before natural weaning age resumed cycling later and suffered a longer inter-birth interval than those whose infants were left with them beyond natural weaning. As such, forced weaning appears to have no appreciable benefit in terms of increased production, possibility the opposite, and this is before taking account of the welfare aspects of the impact on the psychological well-being of the mother or the infant.

The main criterion is the monkeys' well-being and it is important that young monkeys are reared with an appropriate social background. If they are not, then they will show deficiencies in social behaviours. Indicators of poor welfare would include:

- a restricted repertoire of behaviours
- an abnormal activity pattern
- inadequate social behaviour
- abnormal behaviours such as self-injury.

Critically relevant is that monkeys raised without the appropriate social stimulation develop to be dysfunctional in their reproductive behaviour (Goldfoot 1977). Goy *et al.* (1974) report that socially deprived male rhesus do not develop the full double foot-clasp mating stance adopted by undeprived animals, and there will be a higher rate of rejection of infants in primiparous socially deprived females (Suomi 1986).

Batch weaning can be carried out at a regular colony health screen. The juvenile can be marked for identification, its weight and body measurements recorded, and its parents' identities recorded (for a review of marking techniques see Honess & Macdonald 2003). Standard marking in captive populations is through microchipping, coupled with a tattoo of the animal's name or a suitable abbreviation. If required, a blood sample may be taken for screening and a full clinical examination should be carried out by the veterinary surgeon and any deviations from normal recorded and investigated. Any necessary vaccination programme can be started at this time. Weaned animals should be placed in a group together. If there are too many to form just one group, care must be taken not to split up half siblings at this stage. The post-weaned animals should be caught by hand and weights recorded at least monthly.

BREEDING LIFESPAN

Cessation of breeding in wild populations is frequently determined by the lifespan of the species, as death (from disease, parasites, predation, fighting or a basic inability to feed sufficiently) is likely to occur before any biological reproductive senescence occurs. In harem or multimale systems males may breed as long as they retain the required social status to maintain reproductive access to females, and females may breed as long as they are able to achieve the necessary breeding condition (energetic and hormonal). The role of aging in reproductive senescence has been the subject of much research, and much of this in non-human primates has focused on the rhesus macaque (*Macaca mulatta*) (Hendrickx & Dukelow 1995a). There is no evidence for the existence of a menopause in New World primates and they appear to continue breeding, albeit with reduced frequency as they get older, well into old age with lifespans of typically

10–20 years (higher in some species: 40–45 years in *Cebus* sp. and 30–35 years in *Ateles* sp.) (Hendrickx & Dukelow 1995a).

In macaques menopause, including stopping of the menstrual cycle and ovulation, has been determined to be at about 25–30 years and may be accompanied by appearance changes, such as changes in face coloration and a greying and thinning of the hair (Hendrickx & Dukelow 1995a). In addition to changes in the reproductive physiology and anatomy, postmenopausal changes may occur, for example to the skeletal and cardiac system, though it is known that the reproductive lifespan of the female rhesus can be up to 25 years of age (Hendrickx & Dukelow 1995a). Although in male macaques there is no decrease in testosterone levels, there does appear to be a drop-off of reproductive behaviour in older males that is likely to be a result of changes in the central nervous system (Hendrickx & Dukelow 1995a).

Although an aging individual may have ceased to breed frequently (there may even be an increase in the number of stillbirths in older females) this does not mean that this animal does not perform an extremely valuable social role within the group in which it lives. In captive populations the negative effects of the unnecessary removal of older animals may be twofold:

- loss of a socially important individual and any role they may play in educating younger members of the group (e.g. in parenting)
- social perturbation (and hence stress) caused by removing a socially influential older animal – this is particularly true of the removal of older, high ranking females in matrilineal macaque societies.

The periodic change of the resident, breeding male, is a natural part of harem and multimale groups such as are found in macaques and this will also help to maintain breeding production – avoiding boredom with their partner that may occur in the females. However, the removal (particularly culling) of older females from their group should be avoided unless there are over-riding animal health concerns. In the interests of the animal's health and welfare it may be appropriate to embark upon a course of contraception for females that are older and experience problems (e.g. frequent stillbirths), but it is also important for their welfare that they be allowed to remain with their social group.

SELECTION OF BREEDING MALES

Where primates are being bred in captivity and there are sufficient animals available, it may be desirable to select animals for breeding based on aspects of their behaviour, such as their temperament, or their genetic profile. In zoos and wildlife parks stud-book information enables the careful management of captive populations to maximise genetic diversity and minimise the potential negative effects of inbreeding. Breeding facilities that aim to supply animals for research may consider it desirable to place more emphasis on breeding animals that may be placid, curious and amenable to training as well as those that have a specific genetic profile. The tracking of the performance of animals during training both within and upon leaving the breeding facility will help to identify those individuals that produce placid, curious offspring that are more likely to be easily trainable and to cooperate with research protocols. This will contribute, when coupled with the highest welfare standards in housing and husbandry, to a reduction in the stress of primates maintained for research.

Sufficient out-breeding will help to avoid some hereditary conditions or familial predispositions to diseases such as metabolic bone disease (Wolfensohn 2003). In addition researchers working in immunology may require animals of a specific type of major histocompatability complex (MHC), e.g. mamu positive. The MHC is a vital part of the immune system and those individuals with a greater variety of MHC alleles will have more protection from a corresponding diversity of possible diseases (Strier 2000). It would, however, be a mistake to attempt to compose breeding groups of the same MHC type in an effort to produce offspring of a uniform MHC type. Knapp *et al.* (1996) demonstrated, in pig-tailed macaques (*Macaca nemestrina*), that mates sharing the same MHC type suffered significantly more spontaneous abortions (more than 70% of which were attributable to shared parental MHC) than those with different MHC types. This work provides additional support for the important role of the olfactory recognition of MHC type among animals (Brown & Eklund 1994) in avoiding this kind of reproductive wastage while at the same time maximising MHC allele diversity.

FURTHER READING

Abbott, D.H. (1988) Natural suppression of fertility. *Symposium of the Zoological Society of London*, **60**, 7–28.

Abbott, D.H. (1989) Social suppression of reproduction in primates. In: *Comparative Socioecology: The Behavioural Ecology of Humans and Other Mammals* (eds V. Standen & R.A. Foley), pp. 285–304. Blackwell Science, Oxford.

Abbott, D.H., Saltzman, W., Schultz-Darken, N.J. & Tannenbaum, P.L. (1998) Adaptations to subordinate status in female marmoset monkeys. *Comparative Biochemistry and Physiology, Part C*, **119**, 261–274.

Altmann, J. (1980) *Baboon Mothers and Infants*. University of Chicago Press, Chicago, Illinois.

AZA [American Zoo and Aquarium Association] Contraception Advisory Group (2003) Recommendations. http://www.stlzoo.org/downloads/CAGRecommendations2003.pdf

Baker, J.V., Abbott, D.H. & Saltzman, W. (1999) Social determinants of reproductive failure in male common marmosets housed with their natal families. *Animal Behaviour*, **58**, 501–513.

Baskerville, M. (1999) Old World monkeys. In: *The UFAW Handbook on the Care and Management of Laboratory Animals*, (ed. T.B. Poole), 7th edn, pp. 611–635. Blackwell Science, Oxford.

Bateman, A.J. (1948) Intra-sexual selection in *Drosophila. Heredity*, **2**, 346–349.

Brown, J.L. & Eklund, A. (1994) Kin recognition and the major histocompatability complex: An integrative review. *American Naturalist*, **143**, 435–461.

Canfield, D., Brignolo, L., Peterson, P.E. & Hendrickx, A.G. (2000) Conjoined twins in a rhesus monkey (*Macaca mulatta*). *Journal of Medical Primatology*, **29**, 427–430.

Clutton-Brock, T.H. (1988) Introduction. In: *Reproductive Success: Studies of Individual Variation in Contrasting Breeding Systems*. (ed. T.H. Clutton-Brock), pp. 1–6. The University of Chicago Press, Chicago.

Dede, J.A. & Plentl, A.A. (1966) Induced ovulation and artificial insemination in a rhesus colony. *Fertility and Sterility*, **17**, 757–764.

Dixson, A.F. (1998) *Primate Sexuality: Comparative Studies of the Prosimians, Monkeys, Apes and Human Beings*. Oxford University Press, Oxford.

Dukelow, W.R. & Clemens, L.G. (1999) Nonhuman primate *in vitro* fertilization applications to toxicology. In: *Reproduction in Nonhuman Primates: A Model System for Human Reproductive Physiology and Toxicology* (eds G.F. Weinbauer & R. Korte), pp. 151–161. Waxmann Münster, New York.

Dunbar, R.I.M. (1987) Demography and reproduction. In: *Primate Societies*, (eds B.B. Smuts, D.L. Cheney, R.M. Seyfarth, R.W. Wrangham, & T.T. Struhsaker), pp. 240–249. Chicago University Press, Chicago.

Dunbar, R.I.M. (1995) The mating system of callitrichid primates: II. The impact of helpers. *Animal Behaviour*, **50**, 1071–1089.

Fraser, H.M. & Lunn, S.F. (1999) Nonhuman primates and female reproductive medicine. In: *Reproduction in Nonhuman Primates: A Model System for Human Reproductive Physiology and Toxicology*, (eds G.F. Weinbauer and R. Korte), pp. 27–59. Waxmann Münster, New York.

Goldfoot, D.A. (1977) Rearing conditions which support or inhibit later sexual potential of laboratory-born rhesus monkeys: hypotheses and diagnostic behaviours. *Laboratory Animal Science*, **27**, 548–556.

Gomes, D.F. & Bicca-Marques, J.C. (2003) An inversion in the timing of reproduction of captive *Macaca mulatta* in the southern hemisphere. *Laboratory Primate Newsletter*, **42**(4), 6.

Goo, G.P. & Fugate, J.K. (1984) Effects of weaning age on maternal reproduction and offspring health in rhesus monkeys (*Macaca mulatta*). *Laboratory Animal Science*, **34**, 66–69.

Gould, K.G. & Martin, D.E. (1986) Artificial insemination in nonhuman primates. In: *Primates: The Road to Self-sustaining Populations* (ed. K. Benirschke), pp. 425–443. Springer-Verlag, New York.

Goy, R.W., Wallen, K. & Goldfoot, D.A. (1974) Social factors affecting the development of mounting behaviour in male rhesus monkeys. In: *Reproductive Behaviour* (eds W. Montagna and W.A. Sadler), pp. 223–247. Plenum Publishing, New York.

Harcourt, A.H. (1987) Dominance and fertility among female primates. *Journal of Zoology, London*, **213**, 471–487.

Harlow, H.F., Dodsworth, R.O. & Harlow, M.K. (1965) Total social isolation in monkeys. *Proceedings of the National Academy of Sciences*, **54**, 90–97.

Hendrickx, A.G. & Dukelow, W.R. (1995a) Reproductive biology. In: *Nonhuman Primates in Biomedical Research: Biology and Management* (eds T.B. Bennett, C.R. Abee & R. Hendrickson), pp. 365–374. American College of Laboratory Animal Medicine Series. Academic Press, San Diego, California.

Hendrickx, A.G. & Dukelow, W.R. (1995b) Breeding. In: *Nonhuman Primates in Biomedical Research: Biology and Management* (eds T.B. Bennett, C.R. Abee & R. Hendrickson), pp. 147–191. American College of Laboratory Animal Medicine Series. Academic Press, San Diego, California.

Hendrickx, A.G., Peterson, P.E., Otianga-Owiti, G.E., *et al.* (1999) Endocrine and morphological biomarkers of early pregnancy loss in macaques. In: *Reproduction in Nonhuman Primates: A Model System for Human Reproductive Physiology and Toxicology* (eds G.F. Weinbauer & R. Korte), pp. 111–135. Waxmann Münster, New York.

The Home Office Code of Practice for the Housing and Care of Animals used in Scientific Procedures. HMSO, London.

Honess, P.E. & Macdonald, D.W. (2003) Marking and radiotracking primates. In: *Field and Laboratory Techniques in Primatology* (eds J.M. Setchell & D.J. Curtis), pp. 158–173. Cambridge University Press, Cambridge.

IPS (1993) *International Guidelines for the Acquisition, Care and Breeding of Non-human Primates. Primate Report*, Special Issue, International Primatological Society.

Janson, C.H. & van Schaik, C.P. (2002) Ecological risk aversion in juvenile primates: Slow and steady wins the race. In: *Juvenile Primates: Life History, Development, and Behavior* (eds M.E. Pereira & L.A. Fairbanks), pp. 57–74. University of Chicago Press, Chicago, Illinois.

Kirkwood, J.K. & Stathatos, K. (1992) *Biology, Rearing and Care of Young Primates.* Blackwell Science, Oxford.

Knapp, L.A., Ha, J.C. & Sackett, G.P. (1996) Parental MHC antigen sharing and pregnancy wastage in captive pig-tailed macaques. *Journal of Reproductive Immunology*, **32**, 73–88.

Krebs, J.R & Davies, N.B. (1993) *An Introduction to Behavioural Ecology*, 3rd edn. Blackwell Science, Oxford.

Lee, P.C. (1987) Nutrition, fertility and maternal investment in primates. *Journal of Zoology, London*, **213**, 409–422.

Lee, P.C. (1988) Ecological constraints and opportunities: Interactions, relationships, and social organization of primates. In: *Ecology and Behaviour of Food-Enhanced Primate Groups*, Monographs in Primatology, Vol. 11 (eds J.E. Fa & C.H. Southwick), pp. 297–311. Alan R. Liss, New York.

Lee, P.C. (1994) Social structure and evolution. In: *Behaviour and Evolution* (eds P.J.B. Slater & T.R. Halliday), pp. 266–303. Cambridge University Press, Cambridge.

Lee, P.C. (1999) Comparative ecology of postnatal growth and weaning among haplorhine primates. In: *Comparative Primate Socioecology* (ed. P.C. Lee), pp. 111–136. Cambridge University Press, Cambridge.

Marx, P.A., Spira, A.I., Gettie, A., *et al.* (1996) Progesterone implants enhances SIV vaginal transmission and early virus load. *Nature Medicine*, **2**, 1084–1089.

Mendoza, S.P., Lowe, E.L., Resko, J.A. & Levine, S. (1978) Seasonal variation in gonadal hormones and social behaviour in squirrel monkeys. *Physiological Behaviour*, **20**, 515–522.

Morrell, J.M., Nowshari, M., Rosenbusch, *et al.* (1997) Birth of offspring following artificial insemination in the common marmoset, *Callithrix jacchus. American Journal of Primatology*, **41**, 37–43.

Morrell, J.M., Nubbemeyer, R., Heistermann, M., *et al.* (1998) Artificial insemination in *Callithrix jacchus* using fresh or cryopreserved sperm. *Animal Reproduction Science*, **52**, 165–174.

NRC (1997) *The Psychological Well-being of Non-human Primates.* National Research Council, National Academy Press, Washington D.C.

Poole, T.B. (ed.) (1999) *The UFAW Handbook on the Care and Management of Laboratory Animals*, 7th edn. Blackwell Science, Oxford.

Pope, C.E., Dresser, B.L., Chin, N.W., *et al.* (1997) Birth of a western lowland gorilla (*Gorilla gorilla gorilla*) following *in vitro* fertilization and embryo transfer. *American Journal of Primatology*, **41**, 247–260.

Reinhardt, V. (2002) Artificial weaning of Old World monkeys: benefits and costs. *Journal of Applied Animal Welfare Science*, **5** (2), 149–154.

de Ruiter, J.R. & van Hoof, J.A.R.A.M. (1993) Male dominance rank and reproductive success in primate groups. *Primates*, **34** (4), 513–523.

Sacket, G.P., Bowman, R.E., Meyer, J.S., *et al.* (1973) Adrenocortical and behavioural reactions by differentially raised rhesus monkeys. *Physiological Psychology*, **1** (3), 209–212.

Sainsbury, A.W. (1997) The humane control of captive marmoset and tamarin populations. *Animal Welfare*, **6**, 231–242.

Semple, S. & McComb, K. (2000) Perception of female reproductive state from vocal cues in a mammal species. *Proceedings of the Royal Society of London B*, **267**, 707–712.

Sengupta, J., Dhawan, L., Lalitkumar, P.G.L. & Ghosh, D. (2003) A multiparametric study of the action of mifepristone used in emergency contraception using the rhesus monkey as a primate model. *Contraception*, **68**, 453–469.

Setchell, J.M., Lee, P.C., Wickings, E.J. & Dixson, A.F. (2001) Growth and ontogeny of sexual size dimorphism in the mandrill (*Mandrillus sphinx*). *American Journal of Physical Anthropology*, **115**, 349–360.

van Schaik, C.P. (1983) Why are diurnal primates living in groups? *Behaviour*, **87**, 120–144.

van Schaik, C.P. & Hostermann, N. (1994) Predation risk and the number of adult males in a primate group: a comparative test. *Behavioural Ecology and Sociobiology*, **35**, 261–272.

Schrier, A.M. & Povar, M.L. (1984) Twin stumptailed monkeys born in laboratory. *Laboratory Primate Newsletter*, **23** (3), 18.

Smuts, B.B., Cheney, D.L., Seyfarth, R.M., *et al.* (eds) (1987) *Primate Societies*. Chicago University Press, Chicago, Illinois.

Stammbach, E. (1987) Desert, forest and montane baboons: Multilevel-societies. In: *Primate Societies* (eds B.B. Smuts, D.L. Cheney, R.M. Seyfarth, R.W. Wrangham, & T.T. Struhsaker), pp. 112–120. Chicago University Press, Chicago.

Strier, K.B. (2000) *Primate Behavioural Ecology*. Allyn & Bacon, Boston.

Suomi, S.J. (1986) Behavioural aspects of successful reproduction in primates. In: *Primates: The Road to Self-sustaining Populations*, (ed. K. Benirschke), pp. 331–340. Springer-Verlag, New York.

de Waal, F.B.M. (1989) Dominance style and primate social organization. In: *Comparative Socio-ecology: The Behavioural Ecology of Humans and Other Mammals*, (eds V. Standen & R.A. Foley), pp. 243–263. Special Publication No. 6 of the British Ecological Society. Blackwell Science, Oxford.

Waitt, C., Little, A., Wolfensohn, S., *et al.* (2003) Evidence from rhesus macaques suggests that male colouration plays a role in female mate choice. *Proceedings of the Royal Society of London B*, **270** (S2), 144–146.

Wallis, J. & Valentine, B. (2001) Early vs. natural weaning in captive baboons: The effect on timing of postpartum estrus and next conception. *Laboratory Primate Newsletter*, **40** (1), 10–13.

Wolfensohn, S.E. (2003) Case report of a possible familial predisposition to metabolic bone disease in juvenile rhesus macaques. *Laboratory Animals*, **37**, 139–144.

Wrangham, R.W. (1980) An ecological model of female bonded primate groups. *Behaviour*, **73**, 262–299.

Zehr, J.L., Tannenbaum, P.L., Jones, B. & Wallen, K. (2000) Peak occurrence of female sexual initiation predicts day of conception in rhesus monkeys (*Macaca mulatta*). *Reproduction, Fertility and Development*, **12** (8), 397–404.

Chapter 9
Sourcing and transporting primates

BACKGROUND

Those who care for primates in captivity should be aware that any form of transport may induce stress in a primate. Transport may entail moving an animal around within a facility (between rooms or buildings); short local road transport; long (as much as 24 hours) road transport; or combined transportation by plane (nationally or internationally), ship and road with a total journey time that may exceed 60 hours (Prescott 2001). Full account should be taken of the impact on the animals when carrying out a cost–benefit analysis of obtaining and using animals for scientific procedures.

It has been known for some time that transport, even within a facility, can cause changes in an animal's behaviour and physiology that can be related to stress. However, much of this work is restricted to laboratory rodents (Tuli *et al.* 1995) and livestock species such as pigs (Bradshaw *et al.* 1996), cattle (Palme *et al.* 2000) and goats (Sanhouri *et al.* 1989). Little is known of the effects of transport on non-human primates, though it is suspected that they may be significant (Jones & Jennings 1994; Wolfensohn 1997; Prescott 2001).

Prescott (2001) serves as a comprehensive source on the regulations governing the importation and of primates into the United Kingdom as well as an assessment of transport conditions and recent patterns of importation.

Countries of origin

Few callitrichids are imported into the United Kingdom as, following a shortfall in supply during the 1980s when there was an increase in their use due to a shift from Old World to New World monkeys, a number of commercial and non-commercial breeding colonies were established or expanded resulting in an occasional surplus, particularly of the common marmoset (*Callithrix jacchus*). Common sources of other New World primates (e.g. brown capuchin, *Cebus paella*, and squirrel monkeys, *Saimiri sciureus*) include Guyana and Suriname, where they are native (Prescott, 2001).

Apart from breeding facilities in the country of end-use (primarily the USA and Europe) captive-bred sources of macaques used in research are: China, the Philippines, Mauritius, Indonesia and Israel for long-tailed macaques (*Macaca fascicularis*); and China and Vietnam for rhesus macaques (*M. mulatta*). Over a 6-year period in the 1950s an average of approximately 200,000 wild rhesus were exported per year from India for research projects, including polio vaccine development (Peterson 1989). Following the collapse in the wild population of rhesus macaques in India as a result of this trade, the

Indian Government stopped the export of wild-caught rhesus. There may however now be efforts to establish captive breeding facilities in India for the export of this species.

In recent years a number of primate range states have moved to legislate against the export of their wildlife, including primates. Even where the export of captive-bred representatives of indigenous species is permitted, this is often under a quota system. There has been a history of the export of wild-caught olive baboons (*Papio hamadryas anubis*) from African countries (e.g. Kenya) for research use, but the trade in this species from Tanzania and Ethiopia as well as that of the capuchins and squirrel monkeys from Guyana and Suriname is now subject to CITES export quotas (Prescott 2001).

IUCN Red Data Book and specialist groups

Concerns persist about the acquisition and transport of primates from the wild and there is an ongoing debate about the relative merits of basing breeding colonies in the countries where the end-use of the animals is intended. While most scientific use of primates involves species that have relatively low conservation threat status in the wild, as defined by the World Conservation Union (IUCN) in its Red List of Threatened Species (2000) (www.redlist.org) and Action Plans of IUCN Species Survival Commission's (SSC) regional Primate Specialist Groups (African, Asian, Neotropical and Madagascan/lemur), there may still be substantial damage to wild populations in harvesting animals for export. Individual suffering caused during the capture and holding of wild animals can be high with the attendant risks of death, injury and psychological trauma, even under strict veterinary and welfare supervision (Ancrenaz *et al.* 2003; Honess & Macdonald 2003; Jolly *et al.* 2003). Sourcing from the wild is likely to make populations unsustainable in light of the over-harvesting that is often deemed necessary, because some captured animals may prove unsuitable for scientific use owing to clinical and/or subclinical infections, or some may die before or during shipment. The impact of high levels of harvesting particularly affects primates as their long life-history strategies are reflected in a relatively low reproductive turnover, which limits the ability of populations to recover from heavy or repeated depletion in their numbers.

The proportion of primates being imported into the UK that are wild caught compared with those that are captive bred has diminished in recent years as the Home Office and ethical review process will not permit their use, and as a result captive breeding facilities for the most frequently used species have been established. Attention has now shifted to attempts to reduce the number of first generation animals that are transported with the intention of making the breeding centres self-sustaining, without the need to top-up or expand their breeding populations from the wild. This does, of course, present breeding centre managers with an additional challenge in the genetic management of their colony.

CITES

The Convention on International Trade in Endangered Species of Wild Fauna and Flora (CITES) is the agreement that regulates, among its signatory states, the *international* trade in endangered species; be it the whole organism (live or dead) or any part or product of it (http://www.cites.org). CITES has its own system of categorisation for the conservation threat status of a species, with those in Appendix I being considered the most endangered (and in which trade is only permitted in very exceptional cases). Currently all primates are listed as being in either Appendix I (threatened with extinction) or Appendix II (could become endangered without control of trade). CITES permits must be obtained for all movements (import and export) of CITES listed species between countries signed up to the Convention. The implementation of CITES regulations and the administration of the permit system is carried out by the relevant department of the signatory government, in the UK this is the responsibility of the Department for Environment, Food and Rural Affairs (DEFRA) and in the USA it is the US Fish and Wildlife Service. These CITES management authorities are listed in the IATA Live Animal Regulations (2002). These authorities will require (as in the UK) demonstration that 'the importation would not have a harmful effect on the conservation of the species' and documentary evidence 'that the place of destination is suitably equipped to conserve and care for the specimen concerned' (http://www.ukcites.gov.uk/license/GN9_Primates.doc).

IATA Regulations

The International Air Transport Association (IATA) publishes its Live Animal Regulations annually in several languages (English, Spanish and French) and these lay out minimum conditions for the air transport of live animals. These regulations are drawn up with the consultation of CITES and government authorities who have adopted the regulations. They also comply with European Union and United States animal transport legislation. In addition to detailing container requirements the Live Animal Regulations also give information on subjects such as specific government and carrier regulations, advance arrangements, documentation, marking and labelling, and handling procedures. Additional guidance is given on the relevant authorities in each relevant country to contact concerning CITES and animal health regulation. This resource is therefore a vital reference and guide to all those seeking to transport, or to receive live primates.

Other legislation and guidelines

A range of other regulations exist that may be specific to certain countries, and it is beyond the scope of this book to review all the existing legislation covering the international trade in primates. Though it is important to point out that the international regulation of the trade in and transport of animals is provided by CITES and IATA, guidelines have been drawn up by other organisations to provide specific advice, such as the those issued by the International Primatological Society (IPS) (1993 and currently under revision), which represents the considered opinion of the world's authorities on primates concerning their 'acquisition, care and breeding'. Again these guidelines set minimum standards and conditions that should be applied to the transport of primates. Further guidelines have been drawn up by organisations with specific interests and those involved in transporting primates should make themselves familiar with those that are most relevant. For example guidelines on the transport of those species used in laboratory research have been drawn up by the Laboratory Animal Breeders Association of Great Britain (LABA) and the Laboratory Animal Science Association (LASA) (LABA/LASA, 1993 – currently under revision by the Federation of European Laboratory Animal Science Associations (FELASA)).

Many countries have additional compliance requirements associated with animal transport. For example in the United Kingdom issues concerning the transport of animals are covered by the Animal Health Act 1981: The Welfare of Animals (Transport) Order 1997. Further compliance is required under a separate order of the Animal Health Act 1981: The Rabies (Importation of dogs, cats and other mammals) Order 1974, which details the quarantine requirements for animals imported into the UK (also see Chapter 5).

TRANSPORTATION

Debate exists over the merits of obtaining primates from overseas breeding centres versus national breeding centres. This debate has largely been fuelled by the assumed stress suffered by primates during international air transport (Prescott 2001). To date it has not been possible to conduct an examination of the stress suffered by primates purely as a result of air transport. However, Honess *et al.* (2004) examined the effect on the behaviour of a group of long-tailed macaques (*M. fascicularis*) of international air transport coupled with rehousing from a large, outdoor group cage at a breeding centre to group housing in traditional modular caging in an experimental facility. Significant changes in behaviour were observed that did not return to baseline levels within the first month after the animals' move. In this study it was clear that every effort had been made by the supplier to minimise the effect on the animals including:

- No weaning under 12 months of age
- Siting the centre close enough to the airport to ensure the briefest of road journeys (in China these may be as long as 24 hours and, in contrast, less than 30 min in Israel; Prescott 2001)
- Not catching and boxing animals any earlier than necessary before movement
- Airport/airline security and customs officials in attendance at the time of catching/ boxing to avoid lengthy checks and waiting at the airport
- Animals caught by hand (or could be trained to enter boxes) to avoid the use of a sedative/anaesthetic and the need for monitored recovery
- Young animals paired for shipping with individuals from the same weaning group with which they will have already have established a relationship. This ensures social buffering during stressful events (Vogt *et al.* 1981).

A number of air carriers, particularly in the UK, have been targeted by animal rights groups for their role in the transportation of primates, and many specifically exclude the carriage of primates intended for scientific use (IATA 2002). This has typically resulted in the air leg of the importation of primates into the UK terminating at a nearby European airport with the remainder of the journey being completed by road and sea. This results in a lengthening of the total journey and the imposition of an additional handling event for the animals, both of which are likely to have a negative affect on the welfare of the animals. Broom (2003) provides a concise assessment of the factors during transport that cause poor welfare in large animals and many of these hold true for primates. Among the factors to consider are:

- regulatory requirements
- vehicle design
- route planning
- physical and environmental conditions
- species and individual coping ability
- attitude and skills of handling and transporting staff.

For further general discussion of the relationship between welfare, stress and coping see Broom and Kirkden (2004) and Broom (2001).

Conditioning

All efforts should be made to ensure that animals are in prime condition and health before being transported. Pregnant, very young and very old animals should only be transported where there is no other option and should be given special consideration and veterinary monitoring. Where possible all females of reproductive age that have been in contact with a male should have an ultra-sound scan to test for pregnancy, even if they are carrying a very young infant as some species can become pregnant shortly after parturition.

Familiarising animals with people and handling (see Chapter 7) will help to reduce the stress of capture and the handling necessary for the veterinary examination in preparation for transport. There may also be value in familiarising the animals with their transport container; an identical crate to that in which they will be transported could be introduced to their environment several weeks before the planned transport. Further habituation could be achieved by, for example, feeding the animals treats in the crate. Care should be taken to ensure that the crate is the identical size, shape, colour and texture to that which will be used and that there are no features on the outside or, obviously, the interior of the crate that might injure the animals.

Transport containers

Minimum standards of container size and structure are described by IATA (2002). There are four categories of container (CR31, CR32, CR33 and CR34) for use with primates. The container type to be used depends both on the species being shipped and on whether individuals are to be shipped singly or not. Figure 9.1 shows an IATA CR32 compliant container. Each compartment can hold one small macaque adult or two compatible animals under 2 kg. IATA also defines the dimensions and construction (including building materials) of containers to meet their regulations ensuring sufficient space, suitable perching, ventilation, separation and light for the occupants. The collection of faeces and urine (or spilt water) is also important to ensure hygiene and comfort, and the IATA requirements specify the need to include a waterproof droppings tray in the base of the container.

Figure 9.2 shows a range of non-IATA containers for moving primates. Figure 9.2a shows a wooden container which may be used for transporting larger animals singly for

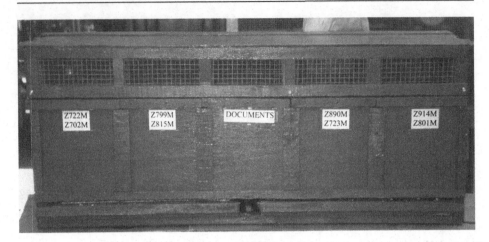

Figure 9.1   An IATA regulation crate used for shipping juvenile (18 month) macaques. Four of the compartments can house two animals each and the central compartment was used for shipping documents.

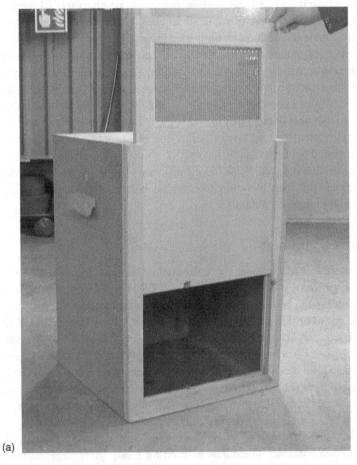

(a)

Figure 9.2   (a) Wooden container used for transporting macaques on short journeys.

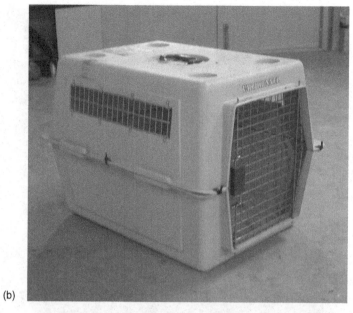

(b)

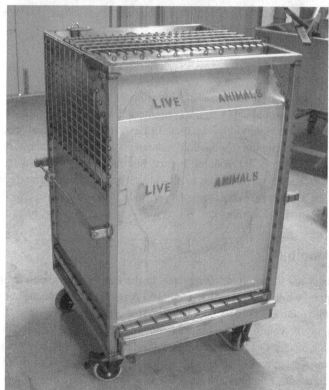

(c)

Figure 9.2   (b) plastic and (c) stainless steel containers used for transporting macaques on short journeys.

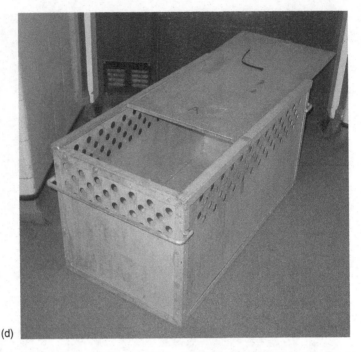

(d)

Figure 9.2   (d) Aluminium containers used for transporting macaques on short journeys.

short journeys only, as it lacks a removable faeces collection tray. The same journey duration restriction would apply to the containers illustrated in Figures 9b–d, which are less suitable for larger individuals as they all have restricted vertical space. The plastic (Figure 9.2b) and aluminium (Figure 9.2d) containers have the advantage over the stainless steel container (Figure 9.2c) in being lighter, but care needs to be taken, with all three and particularly the two metal types, to provide sufficient comfort and thermal insulation with the use of a suitable blanket such as Vet Bed™ (Jørgen Kruuse A/S, Marslev Byvej 35, DK-5290 Marslev, Denmark).

Social groupings

When primates are transported, particularly in the supply of research facilities, they are usually shipped while still juvenile. Under IATA regulation pregnant females and those with suckling young are not accepted for air transport.

The shipping of young animals makes commercial sense as the weight per animal is lower than that of adults and therefore the total weight and resulting cost of the consignment is kept down. An additional advantage is that smaller animals can be shipped in pairs within the transport container. However it is therefore particularly important that the social compatibility of animals transported together should be ensured. Some may worry about the potential for animals to harm each other when subjected to the stressful conditions undoubtedly imposed during the transport process. Evidence suggests that when primates are subjected to a stressful event, either in the presence of conspecifics or when alone, they exhibit markedly reduced physiological stress when in the presence of other individuals. However their behaviour does not necessarily appear to be markedly different (Vogt *et al.* 1981). Pairing animals allows for mutual support during stress. The compatibility of pairings can be ensured by studying the interactions of the animals in the social context in which they are living before being transported; affiliating pairs can then be assigned to travel together. This philosophy should extend beyond the transport phase and efforts should be made to ensure that groups of primates, which are being transported and will be housed together at their destination, are as socially stable as possible and, where possible, from the same breeding group. In this way many of their relationships and their social status will have already been defined in their natal groups, reducing the likelihood and intensity of further conflict. This will therefore make the veterinary and behavioural management of the animals easier.

PROVISION DURING TRANSPORT

Feeding and watering

The IATA Live Animal Regulations (2002) do not require feeding and watering for the 24-hour period after dispatch, however local and regional (e.g. European Union) regulations may require feeding and watering to be more frequent. For this reason, and as a contingency for emergency or delay, food and water that is additional to that supplied to the animals in their compartment of the transport container should be sent with the animals, along with detailed instructions for its use. IATA regulation transport containers are designed to allow access through a well-marked point to food and specifically water containers, which must be entirely housed internally.

As primates can be very selective about their food it is also wise to send with the consignment a sufficient quantity of any familiar, non-perishable/dry diet. This will feed the animals for as long as it takes to source the same diet at the destination, or it will last long enough to wean the animals onto a new diet. Note that a change in diet can affect the gut flora and, with all the other changes involved in transportation, will add to the animals' stress. After a period of dietary consistency, a gradual change to a new diet over 4–5 days will reduce the incidence of diarrhoea. Communication between shipper and recipient, before shipping, should ensure that a list of the animals' favoured and acceptable foods is passed on so that these can be available on arrival.

Environment

The transport environment, whether in an aircraft compartment or the back of a truck or van, is likely to be alien and potentially stressful to all primates. These environments can produce unfamiliar levels of motion, vibration, noise, humidity, temperature and unusual smells. Significant deviation of any of these from those with which they are familiar may have an adverse affect on the welfare of the animals. Climate control (with suitable emergency backup) within these environments is therefore a vital part of reducing the impact of transportation. Good and steady piloting or driving, good container insulation and ventilation, and careful handling will all help minimise the stress placed on the animal. Measures should be taken to prevent exposing the animals to extremes, particularly of temperature or wind/draughts to which primates are particularly sensitive.

Any systematic and objective study of the transport environment and its effect on primates has been limited (Honess *et al*. 2004), and has been frustrated by technological problems as well as limitations imposed by the requirement that any recording equipment on board an aircraft must not interfere with its communication or navigational equipment.

There may also be disease transmission risks associated with the transportation of primates, both between the animals and handling staff and between consignments of animals. Handling staff should take personal hygiene precautions, and transport container design should be such as to prevent physical contact between the animals and staff. This is particularly the case with animals of unknown health profile that may be carrying zoonotic diseases. It also needs to be borne in mind that disease can pass in the other direction; from the handlers to the primates. IATA also points out that primates from different continents should not be shipped together nor should they come into contact at any point during their journey, including on the ground. In addition, shipments of primates destined for laboratories should always be kept away from all other consignments of primates.

POST-MOVE MONITORING

As highlighted at the beginning of this chapter, very little is known about the effect on primates of being transported. It is frequently difficult, if not impossible, to separate the effect of the transport element of their journey from the effect on the animals of other changes that may accompany this: changes in accommodation, animal care staff, diet, climatic conditions etc. Nevertheless changes in a number of aspects of an animal's environment are an integral element in the translocation process and form part of the experience of the animals. The presence of such confounding variables should not therefore deter the assessment of the impact of the total process.

Primates that are transported should receive thorough veterinary examination both before they are transported and upon arrival at their destination. Detailed analysis of the effect on reproduction has also been undertaken: it has been shown that the stress involved in moving a primate colony can have a serious impact on its productivity for an extended period, both in terms of survivorship and disruption to breeding (e.g. delay of maturation in pubescent animals) (Ha *et al*. 2000).

It is rare, however, that transported primates receive a similar level of monitoring of their behaviour. It is easy to detect behaviour that indicates substantial problems, such as self-harming or stereotypic behaviours like circling or saluting, but more subtle behavioural changes, which may be an early indication of stress, are more difficult to detect. Honess *et al*. (2004) examined the behavioural changes in a group of eight juvenile male long-tailed macaques (*Macaca fascicularis*) shipped by air to the United Kingdom from Israel. Assessment of change must by definition include some measurement of the pre-existing state before the change in the animals' circumstances. This study, which may act as a model for further work, was conducted with the full cooperation of the breeding centre management as part of their general consideration for the welfare of the animals they supply. There were considerable differences in the way the animals were housed at their origin and destination, largely due to UK Department of the Environment, Food and Rural Affairs (DEFRA) quarantine regulations and Home Office Code of Practice guidelines for a laboratory environment. These differences were described and quantified, and standardised and objective measures of the animals' behaviour were made, by the same observer, both before (as a baseline) and after the movement. Focal animal sampling (Altmann 1974) was used as it provided the best resolution on individual differences. A range of behaviours were included to enable the detection of changes in the animals' activity patterns and behavioural repertoire as well as to inform about quantified changes in specific behaviours. The dominance hierarchy of the animals was also examined (Martin & Bateson 1993), using a feeding trial, for any change over the study that may reflect social perturbation (see Figure 9.3). Significant differences were found in the activity patterns of the study animals, which indicated increased stress. Post-move changes were examined by repeating the assessment 1 month after the animals' arrival in addition to immediately after arrival. After initial changes noted in the animals' behaviour after arrival it was clear that, despite some adjustment, there was no return within the following month to the behavioural patterns observed at the breeding facility.

Further work of this nature needs to be conducted on a routine basis as part of the continuing assessment of the welfare of primates held in captivity. It will also enable the identification of specific behaviours, changes in which provide the best early indication of compromised animal welfare, and allow planning for the alleviation of the stress under which this places the animals. For efficient, rigorous and objective studies of this type it is important that a professional primatologist is involved in planning. Perhaps with the increasing requirement that primate facilities include a primatologist in their staff, the objective study of the welfare of captive primates will become more commonplace.

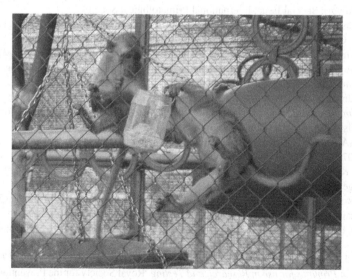

Figure 9.3   Assessing dominance hierarchy using a feeding trial.

FURTHER READING

Altmann, J. (1974) Observational study of behaviour: Sampling methods. *Behaviour*, **49**, 227–267.

Ancrenaz, M., Setchell, J.M. & Curtis, D.J. (2003) In: *Field and Laboratory Techniques in Primatology* (eds J.M. Setchell & D.J. Curtis), pp. 122–139. Cambridge University Press, Cambridge.

Animal Health Act 1981: *Rabies Control Order 1974 and the Rabies (Importation of Dogs, Cats and Other Mammals) Order 1974 and the Welfare of Animals (Transport) Order 1997*. HMSO, London.

Bradshaw, R.H., Parrott, R.F., Goode, J.A., *et al.* (1996) Behavioural and hormonal responses of pigs during transport: effect of mixing and duration on journey. *Animal Science*, **62**, 547–554.

Broom, D.M. (2001) Coping, stress, and welfare. In: *Coping with Challenge: Welfare in Animals including Humans* (ed. D.M. Broom), pp. 1–9. Dahlem University Press, Berlin.

Broom, D.M. (2003) Causes of poor welfare in large animals during transport. *Veterinary Research Communications*, **27** (1), 515–518.

Broom, D.M. & Kirkden, R.D. (2004) Welfare, stress, behaviour, and pathophysiology. In: *Veterinary Pathophysiology* (eds R.H. Dunlop & C-H. Malbert), pp. 337–369. Blackwell Publishing, Ames, Iowa.

Ha, J., Robinette, R. & Davis, A. (2000) Survival and reproduction in the first two years following a large-scale primate colony move and social reorganisation. *American Journal of Primatology*, **50**, 131–138.

The Home Office Code of Practice for the Housing and Care of Animals used in Scientific Procedures. HMSO, London.

Honess P., Johnson P. & Wolfensohn S. (2004) A study of behavioural responses of non-human primates to air transport and re-housing. *Laboratory Animals*, **38**, 119–132.

Honess P. & Macdonald D. (2003) Marking and radio-tracking primates. In: *Field and Laboratory Methods in Primatology: A Practical Guide* (eds D. Curtis & J. Setchell), pp. 158–173. Cambridge University Press, Cambridge.

IATA (2002) *Live Animal Regulations*, 29th edn. International Air Transport Association, Montreal, Canada.

IPS (1993) *International Guidelines for the Acquisition, Care and Breeding of Nonhuman Primates*. *Primate Report*, Special Issue, International Primatological Society.

IUCN Species Survival Commission (2000) *2000 IUCN Red List of Threatened Species*. International Union for Conservation of Nature and Natural Resources, Gland, Switzerland.

Jolly, C.J., Phillips-Conroy, J.E. & Muller, A.E. (2003) Trapping primates. In: *Field and Laboratory Techniques in Primatology* (eds J.M. Setchell & D.J. Curtis), pp. 110–121. Cambridge University Press, Cambridge.

Jones, B. & Jennings, M. (1994) *The Supply of Non-human Primates for Use in Research and Testing: Welfare Implications and Opportunities for Change*. Royal Society for the Prevention of Cruelty to Animals (RSPCA), Horsham, West Sussex, UK.

LABA/LASA (1993) Guidelines for the care of laboratory animals in transit. *Laboratory Animals*, **27**, 93–107.

Martin, P. & Bateson, P. (1993) *Measuring Behaviour: An Introductory Guide*, 2nd edn. Cambridge University Press, Cambridge.

Palme, R., Robia, C., Baumgartner, W. & Möstl, E. (2000) Transport stress in cattle as reflected in faecal cortisol metabolite concentrations. *Veterinary Record*, **146** (4), 108–109.

Peterson, D. (1989) *The Deluge and the Arc: A Journey into Primate Worlds*. Hutchinson Radius, London.

Prescott, M.J. (2001) *Counting the Cost: Welfare Implications of the Acquisition and Transport of Non-human Primates for use in Research and Testing*. Royal Society for the Prevention of Cruelty to Animals (RSPCA), Horsham, West Sussex, UK.

Sanhouri, A.A., Jones, R.S. & Dobson, H. (1989) The effects of different types of transportation on plasma cortisol and testosterone concentrations in male goats. *British Veterinary Journal*, **145**, 446–450.

Tuli, J.S., Smith, J.A. & Morton, D.B. (1995) Stress measurement in mice after transportation. *Laboratory Animals*, **29**, 132–138.

Vogt, J.L., Coe, C.L. & Levine, S. (1981) Behavioural and adrenocorticoid responsiveness of squirrel monkeys to a live snake: is flight necessarily stressful? *Behavioural and Neural Biology*, **32** (4), 391–405.

Wolfensohn, S.E. (1997) Brief review of scientific studies of the welfare implications of transporting primates. *Laboratory Animals*, **31**, 303–305.

Index